Finding
Your Way
to Wellness

Finding Your Way to Wellness

Second Edition

Puget Sound Breast Cancer
Information & Resource Guide

The Susan G. Komen
Breast Cancer Foundation
• Puget Sound Affiliate •

Finding Your Way to Wellness

Second Edition

AUTHORS

Julie Gralow

Denice Bowls
Alice Burgess
Julia Cañas
Kim Dammann
Pat Dawson
Debra Forman
Susan Goedde
Dan Labriola
Elizabeth Landrum
Barbara Lees

Alison Longley
Stephanie Martin
Patti McConnell
Janet Parker
Marisa Perdomo
Martha Purrier
Kate Rose Kilpatrick
Sandra Saffle
C.J. Taylor
Elizabeth J. White

Printed in the United States of America

ISBN 0-9674187-0-4
Second Printing
00-105851
CIP

Cover:
Joan Bowman, "The Big Stretch," wood etching

Published by The Susan G. Komen Breast Cancer Foundation
Puget Sound Affiliate
1900 Northlake Way, Suite 237
Seattle, WA 98103
(206) 633-0303
www.komenseattle.org

❧

*This book is dedicated to all the women
who feel alone as they face the biggest
challenge of their lives: breast cancer.*

*Many have walked before you — and found
their way to wellness. Many walk beside
you — and offer their hands and hearts.*

*Take their hands, open your heart.
And you will not walk alone.*

❧

Kate Rose Kilpatrick

❧

For additional information about
breast health or breast cancer,
call the Komen Foundation's
National Toll-Free Helpline:

1-800-I'M AWARE

Acknowledgments

The Puget Sound Affiliate of the Susan G. Komen Breast Cancer Foundation would like to express thanks to the following sponsors and individuals who have made this book possible:

Bristol-Myers Squibb Oncology, Genentech BioOncology, Ortho Biotech, Merck & Company, Inc., U.S. Human Health, Sue Beale, Susan Bradley, Alice Burgess, Jan Imes, Mysti Jones, Darci Livingston, Alison Longley, Pauline Miyata, May Nagasawa, Manpreet Singh, Jan Slawson, Karen Walter.

And a special thanks to Pricilla Johnston for her leadership in creating this book.

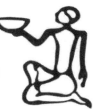

Innervisions:
*Sharing the Journey
of Breast Cancer through
Expressions of Art*

Art by the following artists and writers is part of *Innervisions*, an exhibit by Northwest breast cancer survivors and friends. This exhibit is dedicated to the memory of Julie Wilson Macke.

Kendra Elin Aubin	Sharon Hines-Pinion
Joan Bowman	Lillian Hofflan
Patricia Donlin	Irina Kalendarev
Elizabeth Fischer	Cari Kastama
Elizabeth Halfacre	Kai Leamer

Innervisions is a nonprofit organization, managed by contributing artists. To submit art, make a contribution, or arrange an exhibit, please contact:

Linda Ladzick	or:
224 SW 192nd Street	Alison Longley
Normandy Park WA 98166	Box 85813
(206) 248-1309	Seattle, WA 98145
liljakukka@aol.com	(360) 378-5871 (weekends)

*Innervisions thanks Shurgard Storage
and Daniel Smith Artists' Materials for their support.*

We wish to thank all of those who contributed to the Wall of Hope, a pictorial essay of breast cancer survivors. A selection of contributors is featured in this book.

Table of Contents

(Note: most chapters include a Resources section at the end)

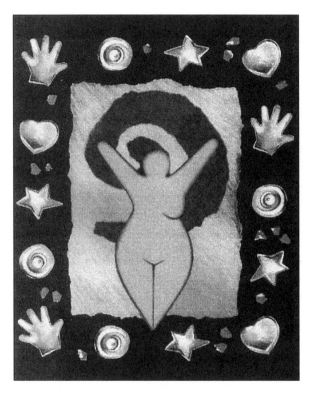

Elizabeth Halfacre ❧ *Survivor* ❧ Pastel & Collage

1

Introduction: The First Step Is Information

ℰℷ

Facing a diagnosis of breast cancer can be overwhelming for patients, their family members and friends. All newly diagnosed patients can benefit from up-to-date information on breast cancer, including how it is diagnosed, what treatment options are available, how to manage treatment side effects, and where to find helpful resources. Recognizing this need, the Puget Sound Affiliate of the Susan G. Komen Breast Cancer Foundation has produced *Finding Your Way to Wellness: The Puget Sound Breast Cancer Information and Resource Guide.*

This is the second edition of *Finding Your Way to Wellness.* Over 12,000 copies of the first edition have been provided to breast cancer patients in the Puget Sound region since 1996. The guide was created in an effort to make information-gathering easier and quicker. This edition includes an overview of breast cancer with references for obtaining further information, as well as listings of resources available to breast cancer patients. The guide was written by a volunteer group of breast cancer survivors and health care professionals in the Puget Sound area. The Susan G. Komen Breast Cancer Foundation does not endorse specific organizations or resources listed in this guide.

It is our hope that this guide will help you through the challenging journey that follows a diagnosis of breast cancer. In order to keep updated on new information, programs, treatments, and research options within the field of breast cancer, we encourage readers to communicate with their health care team, and to contact the Susan G. Komen Breast Cancer Foundation and other breast cancer organizations listed in this guide.

We welcome your feedback, as well as suggestions for resources and information to be included in future editions of this book. Should you have updates, comments or corrections, please contact the Puget Sound Affiliate of the Susan G. Komen Breast Cancer Foundation at (206) 633-0303. Additonal copies of this guide may also be obtained by calling this number.

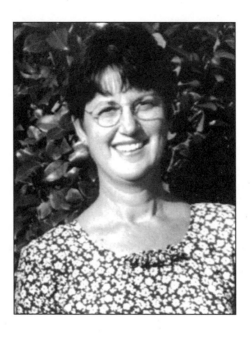

Mary Anne Madsen
Diagnosed: Age 45, 1995

I am celebrating my fourth anniversary of my breast cancer diagnosis, and I am looking forward to September of the year 2000 when I will reach the five-year mark. Because I did practice breast self-exams, I was able to detect a slight change in my breast that felt benign to the professionals but turned out to be cancer. Therefore, my message to women everywhere is: Monthly breast self-exams, regular mammograms, and yearly physical exams could save your life!

2

The Breast Cancer "Epidemic"

Breast cancer is the most common cancer among women. Approximately one in eight women in the United States will be diagnosed with breast cancer in her lifetime. An average woman's chance of getting breast cancer is about one in 200 by age 40, one in 50 by age 50, and one in 25 by age 60. Approximately 80 percent of women with breast cancer in the United States are over age 50, and half of all cases occur in women 65 years and older. Although less common, younger women also get breast cancer.

In 2000, it is estimated by the American Cancer Society that 182,800 women and 1,400 men will be diagnosed with breast cancer in the United States. In Washington state, it is predicted that 3,500 women will be diagnosed with breast cancer in 2000. In the 1980s, breast cancer incidence rates increased by as much as 4 percent per year. This has sometimes been called a breast cancer "epidemic." Most observers, however, consider it to be the result of earlier detection of cancer, thanks to the use of screening mammography. Breast cancer incidence rates have leveled off in the United States in the 1990s at about 110 cases diagnosed per 100,000 women per year.

Although one in eight women in the U.S. will develop breast cancer, only one in 30 will die from this disease. The American Cancer Society estimates that 40,800 women and 400 men will die from breast cancer in 2000. Although there is some fluctuation in the numbers, it looks as if the death rate from breast cancer fell approximately six percent for white women and rose about one percent in black women. The overall rate for American women has fallen about five percent in recent years. This may be due to earlier detection, better treatment, or both. The five-year survival rate for localized breast cancer has increased from 72 percent in the 1940s to 97 percent today. If the cancer has spread regionally (to the lymph nodes), the 5-year survival rate is 77 percent. For women with distant metastases, this rate is 22 percent. Sixty nine percent of all women diagnosed with breast cancer survive 10 years, and 57 percent survive 15 years.

Research suggests that the death rate from breast cancer could decrease by 30 percent if women aged 50 years and older followed screening mammography guidelines. Early detection of breast cancer gives a woman her best chance for survival.

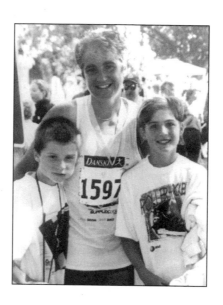

Dana Sigley

Diagnosed: Age 36

I am a very fortunate woman. It has been ten years since my "breast cancer experience." As an operating room nurse and survivor, I give talks about surgery for breast cancer to education/support groups at Swedish Tumor Institute. I am often called upon by friends to speak with women newly diagnosed with this disease. I have met the most amazing women, who have such a variety of stories to tell. I celebrate each of these women I've had the privilege to know. In her March 1993 article, *The Gifts of Cancer?*, Linda Ellerby said, "Look, let's be plain. Having cancer sucks. Chemotherapy was a real drag, surgery was painful, and given a choice, I would prefer having breasts, but my life is better now than it was before cancer. And that's the truth. So, I don't feel like a survivor. I feel like a VICTOR." To that I say, "Amen, sister!"

3

Breast Cancer Risk Factors, Genetics and Prevention

⁊⊋

The development and progression of breast cancer are the result of several mutations or alterations in the DNA of normal breast tissue. It's still not clear what causes the DNA changes that lead to breast cancer, or how to prevent them from occurring. The development of breast cancer appears to be due to a combination of many factors. Researchers are investigating the possible roles of heredity, lifestyle, environment, hormones, and diet.

Gender and Age: The two most significant risk factors for developing breast cancer are being a woman and getting older. Three-quarters of all breast cancers occur in women over age 50. In the U.S., the average age of breast cancer diagnosis is 68 years.

Pregnancy and Menstrual History: Women who have never had children, or had their first child after age 30, seem to be at somewhat higher risk for breast cancer. Women who began menstruating at an early age (before 12) or continued menstruating until a later age (after 55) are also at a slightly greater risk of developing the disease. This is likely due to longer exposure to monthly cycling of the hormone estrogen, which can stimulate normal breast cells to grow.

Hormone Replacement Therapy (HRT) and Oral Contraceptives: The relationship between the hormone estrogen and the risk of developing breast cancer is not well understood. Some studies suggest that long-term use (10 years or more) of HRT for relief of menopausal symptoms may slightly increase the risk of breast cancer. A women's breast cancer risk declines over time once the woman stops taking hormone replacement therapy. There is no clear contraindication to oral contraceptives or HRT in a woman with a family history of breast cancer. However, this area is controversial and studies are still ongoing. In women who have already been diagnosed with breast cancer, some doctors are concerned that the exposure to estrogen will increase a woman's risk of breast cancer recurring.

Studies on breast cancer risk and oral contraceptives are still ongoing, but results have largely shown that oral contraceptive use slightly increases breast cancer risk. No increased risk is associated with taking birth control pills ten years after stopping them.

Environmental Risk Factors: Some suspected breast carcinogens include chlorinated hydrocarbons such as the pesticide DDT, which acts as an estrogen in the body, and ionizing radiation, as from nuclear power plant emissions and high-dose radiation treatment. The benefit from properly performed, low-dose mammography screening greatly outweighs the risk of this minimal radiation exposure.

Benign Breast Disease: Most breast abnormalities do not represent an increased risk of breast cancer, although some are believed to represent precancerous lesions. Most fibrocystic changes, fibroadenomas and cysts do not increase a woman's chances of developing breast cancer. Changes called "atypia" or "hyperplasia" can indicate an increased risk of later developing the disease. This diagnosis can only be made by a pathologist as a result of a breast biopsy. Lobular carcinoma in situ, a precancerous lesion, is associated with a significantly increased risk of the future development of breast cancer.

Exercise: Some studies suggest that exercise may have a protective effect against breast cancer. Recent research has shown that women under 40 who exercise 4 or more hours per week have a lower risk of developing the disease. Exercise reduces the levels of estrogen in the body, and it is thought that estrogen in excess may increase breast cancer risk.

Diet: Obesity, low intake of fruits and vegetables, and high alcohol intake have all been implicated in increasing breast cancer risk. There may be a link between being overweight and a higher risk of breast cancer, especially for women over 50. Studies of fat in the diet as it relates to breast cancer have produced conflicting results. Several studies of women in the U.S. have not found breast cancer risk to be related to fat in the diet. However, there is evidence that the disease is less common in countries where the typical diet is low in fat.

Good general recommendations for a healthy diet that may reduce the risk of developing breast cancer (or prevent its recurrence) include:

- Take off excess weight.
- Minimize the amount of red meat, saturated fat, salt, and sugar.
- Eat a balanced diet with a good variety of nutrients and plenty of fiber—this means plenty of fruits and vegetables!
- If you drink alcohol, do so only in moderation.

Family History and Genetics: Most women diagnosed with breast cancer have a negative family history for the disease. The risk of breast cancer is known to be somewhat higher in women whose close female relatives have had the disease. This risk appears to increase when family members develop breast cancer at a younger age, develop cancer in both breasts, or are more closely related. Breast cancer in two or more family members may increase risk. When looking at family history, it is important to realize that both the maternal (mother's) and paternal (father's) side of the family are equally important.

Of all women with breast cancer, about 5-10 percent have a hereditary (inherited) breast cancer-associated genetic mutation. In families with inherited forms of breast cancer, there are typically more than two first-degree relatives (mother, daughter, sister) with breast or ovarian cancer, and the disease occurs at a young age (40s, 30s or even 20s).

Two breast cancer susceptibility genes, BRCA1 and BRCA2, have recently been identified. Other breast cancer genes will undoubtedly be discovered. There is a 50 percent chance that the mutated copy of a BRCA1 or BRCA2 gene carried by a parent will be passed on to a child. Women who inherit a mutated form of BRCA1 or BRCA2 are highly susceptible to breast and ovarian cancers. Women of Ashkenazi Jewish descent, particularly those with a family history of breast or ovarian cancer, have a higher-than-average risk of carrying a mutated form of the BRCA1 or BRCA2 genes. About 60-80 percent of women with BRCA1 or BRCA2 mutations will develop breast cancer by the age of 70. Men and women with a BRCA1 mutation have a slightly higher lifetime risk of developing colon cancer, and men have a higher lifetime risk for prostate cancer.

Women can now undergo genetic testing for alterations in the BRCA1 and BRCA2 genes, to help determine their cancer risk. Serious challenges need to be overcome in determining whom to test and how to use this information clinically. Genetic testing can tell if a woman has these mutated genes, but it cannot predict whether a woman will get breast or ovarian cancer. Genetic testing is expensive and is not covered by all health plans. It is not clear that screening the general population for these genes will be beneficial. A negative test for these two known genes would not mean that a woman could not develop breast cancer due to other genes or risk factors. There are also ethical, legal, social, and insurance issues related to genetic testing that need to be seriously considered before routinely offering and undergoing such testing. People with positive results might not be able to get insurance, or coverage might only be available at a much higher cost. This is not a test for all women; anyone considering undergoing genetic testing needs to carefully weigh the benefits and drawbacks before proceeding.

Breast Cancer Prevention

All of us will agree that, ideally, preventing breast cancer in the first place would be even better than improved early detection and treatment. Current research on how cell changes can lead to cancer and what factors start, promote, and inhibit these changes gives hope that, in the not-too-distant future, we will understand enough about the causes of breast cancer to prevent many cases. Because the development of cancer is a long, multi-step process, there are many ways in which it might be prevented. Avoiding exposure to carcinogens (cancer-causing agents) prevents the first step that leads toward cancer, and is called primary prevention. Most breast cancer prevention research is aimed at secondary or tertiary prevention: stopping the process of cancer development after it has begun.

Several approaches to breast cancer prevention are currently being tested through clinical research. There are studies underway designed to evaluate dietary and lifestyle approaches to breast cancer prevention. Other studies are examining the effectiveness of "chemoprevention"— using chemicals or drugs to reduce breast cancer incidence.

In the United States, a hormonal therapy which is presently used in treatment of breast cancer, tamoxifen (Nolvadex), has been tested as a chemopreventive agent. Because it is known that women who take tamoxifen for breast cancer have fewer second breast cancers, it was suspected that women who do not presently have breast cancer but who are at high risk for developing the disease may have this risk reduced by taking tamoxifen. The National Surgical Breast and Bowel Project's (NSABP) P-01 **Breast Cancer Prevention Trial** compared breast cancer incidence in high-risk women taking tamoxifen for five years with those taking a placebo (a pill containing no medication). This study showed that women at high risk for breast cancer are about 50 percent less likely to develop the disease (at least in the short term) if they take tamoxifen. To date, although the number of breast cancers has been reduced, no improvement in overall survival has been seen in the tamoxifen group.

Tamoxifen has some known toxicities. Endometrial (uterine) cancer, blood clots, strokes, hot flashes, and vaginal discharge all occurred at increased rates in women taking tamoxifen compared to those taking a placebo. It is felt that the benefits of tamoxifen outweigh its risks in women with a high risk of developing breast cancer, but the risks probably outweigh the benefits in women at low to moderate risk. If a woman is at high risk for breast cancer, or for developing a second breast cancer, she should discuss chemoprevention strategies such as tamoxifen with her health care provider.

Raloxifene (Evista) is a newer selective estrogen receptor modulator (SERM), similar to tamoxifen. The major difference between tamoxifen and raloxifene is the effect on the endometrium. Raloxifene does not appear to stimulate the uterine lining, and therefore should not lead to increased endometrial cancers. Raloxifene has been much less thoroughly studied with respect to breast cancer, and currently is approved only for treatment of osteoporosis. The NSABP is conducting a study comparing the breast cancer prevention effects of tamoxifen to those of raloxifene. The **STAR Trial** (Study of Tamoxifen And Raloxifene) is recruiting postmenopausal women with a higher than average risk of breast cancer, including women with a family history of breast cancer in close relatives, some types of benign breast disease requiring biopsies, reproductive and hormonal histories placing them at increased risk, and women who are over 60 years of age. If you are interested in participating in this study or have questions about it, contact Joelle Machia at the Fred Hutchinson Cancer Research Center (206-667-6544).

In Italy, a retinoid called fenretinide (a chemical similar to vitamin A) is being tested in women who have had cancer in one breast to see if their risk of second breast cancers is reduced. Although retinoids can be toxic, there is evidence that they are effective in preventing skin, oral, bladder, and cervical cancers. Preliminary results from the Italian study suggest that it may reduce ovarian cancer, but its effect on second breast cancers has not yet been reported.

In some rare cases, a woman at high risk might consider preventive (prophylactic) mastectomy. This is an operation in which one or both breasts are removed before there is any known breast cancer. The reasons for considering this type of surgery need to be very strong. While the operation reduces the risk of breast cancer, it doesn't guarantee that cancer won't develop in the small amount of breast tissue remaining after the operation. Clearly, this is something a woman should discuss carefully with her health care provider.

There are many unknowns in breast cancer prevention, but we are learning more all the time. Meanwhile, we can act individually to reduce our risks through diet, exercise, and avoidance of unnecessary exposure to carcinogens. Some of us can participate in clinical trials, and all of us can hope to see fewer of our family and friends stricken as we learn how to stop the long process that leads to breast cancer.

℘RESOURCES
Books

Davies, K., and White, M. Breakthrough: The Race to Find the Breast Cancer Gene (John Wiley and Sons, Inc., 1996)

Kemeny, M., and Dranov, P. Breast and Ovarian Cancer: Beating the Odds (Addison-Wesley, 1992)

Eades, M. If It Runs in Your Family: Breast Cancer: Reducing Your Risk (The Philip Lief Group, 1991)

Bennett, R. The Practical Guide to Genetic Family History (John Wiley & Sons, 1999)

Baker, N. Relative Risk: Living with a Family History of Breast Cancer (The Penguin Group, 1992)

Kelly, P. Understanding Breast Cancer Risk (Temple University, 1991)

Publications

National Cancer Institute, Understanding Gene Testing (National Institutes of Health Publication No. 96-3905)
The Cancer Information Service of the National Cancer Institute can be reached via its toll-free number, 800-4-CANCER, or at www.icic.nci.nih.gov

Myriad Genetics Laboratories. Genetic Analysis for Risk of Breast and Ovarian Cancer: Is It Right for You? (1996)
Available at no charge from Myriad 800-469-7423; www.myriad.com

National Action Plan on Breast Cancer, Genetic Testing for Cancer Risk: It's Your Choice
13-minute video and companion brochure. For free copy, write to the National Action Plan on Breast Cancer, PHS Office on Women's Health, 200 Independence Avenue SW, Room 718F, Washington, D.C. 20201

American Jewish Congress and Hadassah, Understanding Genetics of Breast Cancer for Jewish Women (1997)
Available by calling Hadassah Health Education Dept., (212) 303-8094

Local Breast Cancer Genetics and Risk Evaluation Clinics

University of Washington Breast and Ovarian Cancer Genetics Center
Box 357720
Seattle, WA 98195
(206) 616-2135
Contact: Robin Bennett, breast cancer genetics counselor.

Swedish Hospital Medical Center
747 Broadway Ave.
Seattle, WA 98122-4037
(206) 386-2101
Contact: Bob Resta, Deborah Dunne, and Sanda Coe, genetics counselors.

Department of the Army
Madigan Army Medical Center
Breast Cancer Initiative
Cancer Genetics Clinic
Tacoma, WA 98431
Contact: Jamilyn Daniels, Genetic Counselor (253) 968-0786
Sharon Taylor, BCI Administrative Assistant (253) 968-0756

Genetic counseling, education and testing for BRCAI and BRCA2 provided to military beneficiaries

Spokane Genetics Clinic
(509) 473-7115 or 800-945-7115
604 W. 6th Avenue
Spokane, WA 99204

Pacific Northwest Regional Genetics Group — Cancer Subcommittee
Fred Hutchinson Cancer Research Center
1100 Fairview Ave. N., MP 702
P.O.Box 19024
Seattle, WA 98109
(206) 667-7806
Contact: Julie Bars Culver, genetics counselor.

National Resources

Strang Cancer Prevention Center. A free national resource for breast cancer risk counseling and research into breast cancer risk. Strang operates a National High Risk Registry for purposes of research and educating participants. A newsletter is published. 428 East 72nd Street, New York, NY 10021, (800) 521-9356 or (212) 794-4900.

Women at Risk. A research, diagnosis and treatment group for women at high risk of developing breast cancer. Columbia-Presbyterian Medical Center, Breast Service, New York, NY, (212) 305-2500.

Facing Our Risk of Cancer Empowered (FORCE). Website and chatroom for women at risk for breast and ovarian cancer. www.facingourrisk.org

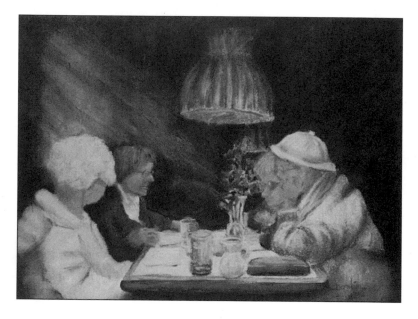

Patricia Donlin ❧ *Still Together, Childhood Friends, Grandma Faces* ❧ Pastel

4

Screening and Diagnosis: Breast Self Exam, Mammography, and Biopsy

ℰ∂

Your best guidelines for a breast health program include the following:

1. Breast Self Exam

Breast Self Exam (BSE) begins with the pads of your fingers, not the nails. Palpate all the breast tissue, including the underarm area. Breasts are the least lumpy and painful at the conclusion of a menstrual cycle. If you are no longer having periods, pick a day of the month and do the exam on the same day each month. A good breast exam includes examining breasts in front of a mirror as well as while lying down. Eighty percent of all breast lumps are found by women themselves AND most are not cancerous.

An important thing to remember about self breast exam is to JUST DO IT!!! Don't be afraid of finding something, or having trouble figuring out what's normal. The more you examine your breasts over time, the more familiar you will become with their contours. Any change should be followed up with your health care provider.

2. Clinical Breast Exam

A thorough exam by your health care provider is recommended for women at least once every three years, beginning at age 20, and annually after age 40.

3. Mammography

The Susan G. Komen Breast Cancer Foundation recommends the following screening guidelines for all women:

- Annual screening mammography for women by age 40.

- Women under 40 with either a family history of breast cancer or other concerns about their personal risk should consult with a trained medical professional about when to begin mammography.

Remember, good breast health includes all three elements: breast self-exam, clinical breast exam, and mammography. This combination gives you the best possible chance of early detection of breast cancer, with the highest likelihood of cure.

Biopsy

If you discover a lump in your breast, you will want to be sure the lump or change is not breast cancer. You may need to have some of the lump removed (a biopsy) so a diagnosis can be made by a pathologist. The pathologist will determine if the tissue removed by the biopsy is normal or cancerous. You will probably have one of the following types of biopsies:

- **Fine needle aspirate** (FNA): A small, thin needle removes a few cells, which are placed on a slide. The pathologist will look for abnormal cells. This may not yield enough information and additional tests may be required. It can be done in the doctor's office and only takes a few minutes.

- **Core needle biopsy**: A larger needle removes a small piece of tissue from the lump. This biopsy is done with local anesthetic in the office or hospital.

- **Surgical biopsy**: The surgeon will remove a portion of the lump or the entire lump. This is scheduled as an out-patient procedure and is done under local anesthesia, with or without sedation.

- **Stereotactic breast biopsies:** This type of biopsy, guided by special mammography machines, can direct a biopsy needle to a specific area of abnormality seen on the scan. Guided biopsies can greatly improve upon the reliability of the tissue sample obtained, and result in reduced trauma to the patient.

New Breast Imaging Techniques

Mammography is an excellent technique for screening and diagnosing breast cancer in most women, but it lacks sensitivity in patients with dense or irregular breasts, particularly younger women. New diagnostic imaging techniques like ultrasound, Magnetic Resonance Imaging (MRI), Computerized Tomography (CT), Positron Emission Tomography (PET) and MIBI (Miraluma) scans are being investigated as supplements to mammography in imaging "difficult" breasts. These tests may increase the detection of small breast cancers and recurrences at an early stage.

✍RESOURCES

Books

McGinn, K.A. The Informed Woman's Guide to Breast Health (Bull Publishing, 1992)

Pamphlets

American Cancer Society. How to Do Breast Self Examination (# 2088-BCN) (800) 227-2345

American Cancer Society. American Cancer Society's Guidelines for the Early Detection of Breast Cancer (# 3304-CC) (800) 227-2345

National Cancer Institute. Are You Over 50? A Mammogram Could Save Your Life (NCI Pub. 93-3418) (800) 624-7890

National Cancer Institute, Questions and Answers about Choosing a Mammogram Facility (NCI Pub. 94-3228) (800) 624-7890

Video

The New BSE: Breast Self Examination by Lange Productions, 1998
To order: 888-LANGE-88

Organizations

Susan G. Komen Breast Cancer Foundation (International Headquarters)
(972) 855-1600
(800) I'M AWARE [(800) 462-9273]
FAX: 972-855-1605
www.breastcancerinfo.com, or www.komen.org

Y-ME National Breast Cancer Organization Hotline
(800) 221-2141
212 W. Van Buren St.
Chicago, Il 60607
(312) 986-8338
www.y-me.org

American Cancer Society
(800) ACS-2345
P.O. Box 142302
Austin, TX 78714-2302
www.cancer.org

National Alliance of BreastCancer Organizations (NABCO)
888-80-NABCO
9 East 37th St., 10th floor
New York, NY 10016
www.nabco.org

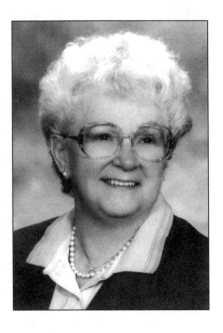

Evelyn Driscoll
Diagnosed: 1990

I am a charter member of an eight-year-old support group, Bosom Buddies, at Evergreen Hospital. I am also considered the unofficial "den mother" of the group because most of the women who have come through the groups are young enough to be my daughters. In our support group, we curse our diagnosis, as well as cry, laugh, and hug to relieve our tensions. "No matter how hard things are, we can handle one day at a time. Yesterday is already a dream and tomorrow is only a vision, but today well lived makes every day yesterday, a dream of happiness and tomorrow a vision of HOPE!"

5

Dealing With A New Diagnosis of Breast Cancer

✄

Learning that you have breast cancer is shocking and terrifying. At first, you may find it hard to control your feelings. You may feel anxious, afraid, sad or depressed. This is normal. Acknowledging and learning how to understand and manage your feelings can help ensure that your emotions don't interfere with your care. Most people feel tremendous loss at the time of diagnosis. You may lose opportunities, your sense of yourself as a healthy person, and your ability to work, if only for a time — resulting in a loss of financial security and independence. The experience of loss, whether actual or anticipated, commonly creates feelings of sadness, depression, anger, fear, anxiety, isolation, loneliness and guilt.

It may help to stop periodically and think about how you are feeling. Some people find that writing in a journal or talking to a trusted friend helps to clarify their emotions. Try to accept your feelings, whatever they are. There is no right or wrong way to feel at such a difficult time. You may be inclined to keep information about your situation to yourself, not wanting to upset or burden your friends and family. It is usually easier on them, however, to know what you are dealing with and how you are really feeling.

Expressing emotions helps us to gradually become more comfortable with them so that they have less influence on our behavior. For example, talking about anger at being ill can eventually enable you to accept that cancer is something that just happened. There is no set reason for it that we can understand, no definite answer to the question, "Why me?" Sharing your thoughts with someone you trust — friend, family member or counselor — can be very comforting. Since those closest to you may feel obligated to offer advice or solutions, you may wish to explain that listening and trying to understand are enough. If you are not able to talk with someone, try writing your feelings down. Expressing yourself verbally or in writing can help you to understand and control your emotions, instead of feeling that they are controlling you.

Maintain a Positive Attitude

Many patients have said that the period before they began treatment was the most difficult. Once you actually start treatment, you may feel better. You begin to get comfortable with your healthcare team and make connections with other patients who are being treated at the same time. You begin to see what the treatment is like and how you are reacting to it. By this time, you will probably have learned about potential problems related to your treatment, which can help you feel more in control.

Because each patient is unique, reactions to treatment — even the same treatment — can vary widely. Some patients have little trouble, while others may experience several problems. You can minimize problems by keeping your medical caregivers informed and by keeping yourself in the best condition possible. Adequate sleep, good nutrition, and appropriate exercise have never been more important. Taking care of yourself emotionally is essential as well.

Try to think positively. You may not be able to choose your reality, but you can choose how to think about and respond to it. Do you see yourself as a helpless victim or as a fighter with a powerful team of doctors, family and friends supporting you? The way you choose to define your situation can have a powerful effect on your outlook.

Thinking positively does not mean ignoring potential threats and dangers; it means choosing not to focus on the negatives of your situation. Focus instead on the reasons you can feel hopeful about your treatment, the knowledge and special skill of your physicians, the support of your family, the good things in your life that you can appreciate right now, your strengths, and your success in solving other problems in your life.

Some patients find spiritual beliefs and prayer helpful in maintaining a positive focus. Others find that relaxation techniques or meditation are powerful tools for regaining focus. Taking a positive approach to situations that arise during your treatment day-to-day can also contribute to your sense of control. And, as with all medical concerns, it is a good idea to anticipate problems that may occur.

Take an Active Role in Your Treatment

Research suggests that people who take an active part in their care and make their own decisions adjust better to major challenges such as a diagnosis of breast cancer.

Begin by establishing good relationships with your doctor(s) and other health care providers. While we tend to assume that all physicians are experienced, attentive, kindly and caring human beings, doctors — like any other group of individuals — may be saints, sinners, jerks or jewels. As in any relationship, communication between patients and their doctors involves give and take. Under the best of circumstances, the communication process evolves into a mutual partnership. Most patients want, at least in part, to make their own care decisions. If this is true for you, let your doctor know that you expect to be a member of your medical team and want to participate in treatment decisions. Some tips for developing effective communication are:

- Decide what kind of doctor(s) you want and seek them out.

- Always ask questions and ask for information to be repeated if it is unclear.

- Write your questions down ahead of time and make sure that all of them are answered. You may want to request descriptions of tests or treatments, information on their benefits and risks, which are recommended and why, and any relevant insurance issues. Ask for another appointment if you need more time. Getting your questions answered can add to your sense of control.

- Keep a notebook and write down notes from meetings with your doctors, names of your care team, medications and dosages, dates of tests, and so on. You will be receiving a great deal of important information, and may find that you need an organizing system to keep track of it all. The resources at the end of this chapter include a book by Swirsky and Balaban which contains appendices including "How to Create a Notebook." Some drug companies produce treatment planners and guides, and many larger treatment facilities provide patient notebooks designed for this purpose. Ask your care team about resources that may be available to you. Local book and stationery stores also carry planners that can easily be adapted.

- Take someone with you to your appointments to be your notetaker, or use a tape recorder so you can review the information again. One person usually cannot hear and absorb all that is said.

• Ask for information to be repeated or stated in more understandable language if it is unclear.

• If you find communication with your doctor is difficult, let him or her know. If this is not comfortable for you, tell another member of your care team whom you find approachable. He or she may be able to help clear up any misunderstandings or suggest strategies for communicating more effectively.

• If communication is still difficult, you may want to consider changing doctors. It is important to find a doctor with whom you communicate well as you enter the treatment process.

Making Decisions

Women have found a variety of tools helpful in making difficult decisions. Some write down their options, listing the pros and cons of each. Others use the more intuitive approaches of meditation, prayer or drawing. Talking to a neutral friend or resource person can also help. (See Resources at the end of this chapter.) Everyone has her own decision-making style. Some women rely primarily on feelings and intuition; others use logic and reason. Some women make decisions quickly, while others need a lot of time to evaluate their options. What is important is to take charge of the process. No matter how you come to your treatment decisions, it is important to make the decision that is right for you. It is natural to feel fearful or uncertain about upcoming surgery, radiation treatment or chemotherapy. If you research and review all your options thoroughly, when you do decide on a treatment you will have more confidence. Standing firmly behind your decision can help to reduce fears and uncertainty and allow you to focus on making the treatment work.

℗RESOURCES

In addition to the treatment information provided by your doctor, local bookstores, libraries, and hospital libraries or resource centers have many resources that address the challenges of coping with a cancer diagnosis, treatment and recovery. Many Internet resources are also now available. If you do use the web for this purpose, make sure that the information you are getting is reliable and trustworthy. Is the source affiliated with a university, health foundation or government health agency? You may want to go exploring on your own or ask your care team for suggestions. Following is a sampling of resources currently available.

Books

Anderson, G. Fifty Essential Things to Do When the Doctor Says It's Cancer (Plume/Penguin Books, 1993)

Harpham, W.S. Diagnosis Cancer: Your Guide through the First Few Months (W.W. Norton & Company, 1998)

Hoffman, B. (ed.) A Cancer Survivor's Almanac: Charting Your Journey (Chronimed Publishing, 1996)

La Tour, K. "It Begins", chapter in The Breast Cancer Companion (Avon Books, 1993)

Leigh, S. "Choice And Decision Making for Women with Breast Cancer" chapter in Dow, K.H. (ed.) Contemporary Issues in Breast Cancer, pp. 143-150 (Jones & Bartlet, 1996)

Morra, M., and Potts E. Triumph: Getting Back to Normal When You Have Cancer (Avon Books, 1997)

Swirsky, J., and Balaban, B. The Breast Cancer Handbook (1994) Contains two useful appendices: "How to Create a Notebook," and "How to Become Your Own Investigative Reporter"

Zakarian, B. The Activist Cancer Patient: How to Take Charge of Your Treatment (John Wiley & Sons, 1996)

Publications

American Cancer Society. Listen with Your Heart
(pamphlet for friends and family of cancer patients, 1996)

American Cancer Society. Talking with Your Doctor
(pamphlet for patients, 1995)

American Cancer Society and National Comprehensive Cancer Network
(NCCN). Breast Cancer Treatment Guidelines for Patients
(Version 1, January 1999)
888-9099-NCCN (www.nccn.org) or 800-ACS-2345
(www.cancer.org)

Coping With Cancer (a bimonthly subscription magazine)
(615) 791-3859 (telephone orders)
P.O. Box 682268
Franklin, TN 37064
E-mail: Copingmag@aol.com

Carries articles on communication, coping with treatment and
survivorship. Many doctors' offices and treatment facilities provide copies
in their patient waiting areas. Unfortunately, "Coping" is not indexed,
making it difficult to identify and access articles.

National Cancer Institute. Understanding Breast Cancer Treatment:
A Guide for Patients (National Institutes of Health Publication No. 98-
4251, 1998)

Videotapes

National Coalition for Cancer Survivorship (NCCS). Cancer Survival
Toolbox: Building Skills that Work for You (1998)

Free set of six self-learning audiotapes which may be listened to
sequentially or individually. Covers communicating, finding information,
making decisions, solving problems, negotiating, and standing up for
your rights.

Organizations

American Cancer Society
800-ACS-2345
P.O. Box 142302
Austin, TX 78714-2302
www.cancer.org

Services include the Reach to Recovery program, Look Good-Feel Better program, general cancer information.

Cancer Lifeline
Dorothy S. O'Brien Center
6522 Fremont Avenue N
Seattle, WA 98103-5358
Program information: (206) 297-2100
24-Hour Lifeline: (206) 297-2500 (King County), or (800) 255-5505 (toll-free in Washington state)
www.cancerlifeline.org

Provides information and referral and phone counseling. Also offers free programs for cancer patients and survivors, their families, coworkers and friends. Workplace consultation for a fee.

Cancer Hope Network
2 North Road, Suite A
Chester, N.J. 07930-2308
877-HOPE-NET (877-467-3638)
www.cancerhopenetwork.org
Nationwide support

One-to-one emotional support for patients and families undergoing chemotherapy and/or radiation treatment, from trained volunteers who have experienced the treatments themselves.

Cancer Information Service
800-4-CANCER (422-6237) (Monday through Friday 9 a.m. to 4:30 p.m. local time)
www.nci.nih.gov (National Cancer Institute)

A program of the National Cancer Institute that provides information on cancer, cancer prevention, publications, community resources, and assistance with cancer education efforts for cancer patients and family members as well as health professionals and others. Services also available in Spanish.

CancerLink
Overlake Hospital Medical Center
1035 116th Avenue N.E.
Bellevue, WA 98004
(425) 688-5266
Patient Education: (425) 688-5248, dbarnes@overlakehospital.org
Voice-mail: (425) 688-5266
E-mail: C-Link@overlakehospital.org
www.overlakehospital.org

Links cancer patients with cancer survivors and family members and caregivers via telephone for confidential one-on-one support

**The Susan G. Komen Breast Cancer Foundation,
Puget Sound Affiliate**
P.O. Box 85900
1900 N. Northlake Way, Suite 237
Office: (206) 633-0303
Fax: (206) 633-0304
E-mail: sgk@pskomen.org
www.komenseattle.org

**The Susan G. Komen Breast Cancer Foundation,
International Headquarters**
5005 LBJ Freeway, Suite 250
Dallas, Texas 75244
(972) 855-1600
Helpline: 800-I'M AWARE
www.breastcancerinfo.com

An international organization with a network of volunteers working through local Affiliates and Komen Race for the Cure® events to eradicate breast cancer as a life threatening disease.

National Alliance of Breast Cancer Organizations (NABCO)
9 East 37th Street, 10th Floor
New York, NY 10016
Office: (888) 806-2226 or (212) 889-0606
Fax: (212) 689-1213
Information Services: (212) 719-0154
www.nabco.org

Membership and advocacy organization of over 300 breast cancer organizations. Provides individualized information package on breast cancer treatment, support services, financial assistance/reimbursement, free or low-cost services, etc. Produces an annual comprehensive listing of national resources, including printed materials, videos, hotlines and a database of support organizations, medical services and advocacy efforts. Quarterly newsletter.

Y-ME
212 West Van Buren St.
Chicago, IL 60607
Hotlines: (800) 221-2141 (24-hours/7 days a week)
(800) 986-9505 (Spanish)
www.y-me.org

Provides presurgical information and referral and phone counseling. Hotline volunteers are breast cancer survivors. Produces several pamphlets ("For Single Women with Breast Cancer," "I Still Buy Green Bananas: Living with Hope, Living with Breast Cancer," etc.) and a bimonthly newsletter with current treatment and clinical trials information.

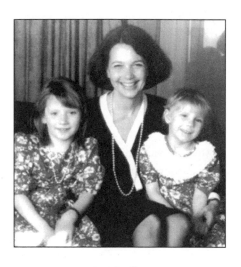

CJ Taylor
Diagnosed: Age 38, 1988

My breast cancer diagnosis did not really come as a surprise to me because my mother died of breast cancer when she was 42. I was 17. I thought I would probably get breast cancer at some point in my life; the only question was when. Luckily, I believed that I could find it early if I had mammograms and checked for lumps. I found my lump. It was discounted by physicians until I had a mammogram six months later. The mammogram showed a small cancer. I have been involved with the Susan G. Komen Breast Cancer Foundation from 1993 to the present, and I have worked at Providence Comprehensive Breast Center. Presently, I am the Executive Director of our Puget Sound Affiliate of the Susan G. Komen Breast Cancer Foundation. I am also an executive council member for Washington state's Breast and Cervical Health Program and a graduate of Project LEAD of the National Breast Cancer Coalition. Please be vigilant so that if you are destined to have breast cancer you, too, will find it early and live a long and productive life. Five years after my diagnosis, my husband, Bob, and I adopted two fabulous daughters. I have a great life.

6

Before Treatment Begins:
Staging, Lab Tests, Second Opinions

ᏯᎯ

Staging

Breast cancer is a disease in which cells that are found in normal breast tissue become malignant, growing and spreading uncontrollably. Breasts are composed of lobules which are connected by thin tubes called ducts. The most common type of breast cancer is ductal cancer. It is found in the cells of the ducts. Cancer that begins in the lobules is called lobular cancer. Lobular cancer is more often found in both breasts (bilaterally) than other types of breast cancer.

The **stage** of breast cancer is a measure of how advanced the cancer is at diagnosis. With increasing use of screening mammograms, breast cancers are diagnosed now at stages earlier than they were previously. The stage of a breast cancer reflects:

- tumor size

- lymph node involvement (whether there is spread through the lymphatic system within the breast to the regional lymph nodes)

- local spread (whether there is spread to neighboring structures like the skin or chest wall)

- distant spread (whether there is metastasis, or spread to distant organs like the lungs, liver or bones, which generally occurs through the lymphatics or bloodstream).

Carcinoma in situ: Stage 0. An abnormal growth of cells that stay within the area in which it started and does not spread is called carcinoma in situ. About 15-20 percent of breast cancers are in situ, or noninvasive. Because it is entirely surrounded by the wall of the duct or lobule, noninvasive breast cancer does not grow into the rest of the breast tissue and does not have access to blood vessels or lymphatics.

There are two types of breast cancer in situ. Ductal carcinoma in situ (DCIS, also known as intraductal carcinoma) arises from the ducts. DCIS is thought to have the potential to develop into an invasive cancer, so it must be treated. Lobular carninoma in situ (LCIS) is not cancer, but for purposes of classifying the disease, it is called breast cancer in situ. Patients with LCIS have a 25 percent chance of developing breast cancer in either breast in the next 25 years. The usual recommendation for women with LCIS is close monitoring and screening.

Early Invasive Breast Cancer: Stages I and II. More than 50 percent of women with invasive breast cancer have stage I disease at diagnosis (a tumor size of 2 centimeters or smaller, without spread to lymph nodes). Another 25 to 30 percent have stage II breast cancers (2 cm or smaller with lymph node involvement, greater than 2 cm and less than 5 cm with or without lymph node involvement, or greater than 5 cm without lymph node involvement). These are often referred to as **early** breast cancers.

Advanced Invasive Breast Cancer: Stages III and IV. Only a minority of patients have stage III (locally advanced) or stage IV (distant spread or metastatic) disease at the time of diagnosis. Inflammatory breast cancer is classified as stage IIIB. It is an uncommon type of cancer in which the breast is warm, red, and swollen due to invasion of tumor into the lymphatics of the skin.

Special Laboratory Tests

Hormone receptor tests for estrogen and progesterone receptors are done on breast cancer tissue removed during biopsy or surgery to help determine prognosis and predict whether the cancer is sensitive to hormone therapy. When the hormones estrogen and progesterone attach to these receptors found in normal breast cells or breast cancer cells, they send a series of signals that can stimulate the cells to grow and divide.

Hormone receptor tests help physicians decide whether hormone therapy or chemotherapy may be useful for a given patient. Positive test results mean that cancer is more likely to respond to hormone treatment, such as the anti-estrogen drug,tamoxifen. Tumors that have hormone receptors are generally associated with a more favorable prognosis.

Paradoxically, breast cancers in women who are post-menopausal are more likely to have positive hormone receptors than are those in pre-menopausal women.

Other tests on breast cancer tissue are sometimes done to help predict whether the tumor is likely to grow slowly or quickly, whether it is likely to recur, and which treatments are likely to be effective. These tests might include **oncogene** or **tumor suppressor gene** tests,which look for mutations in cancer-related genes and proteins including HER-2 (C-erb B-2 or HER-2/neu) and p53. **Measurements of cell proliferation or DNA content** may include **Ki67**, S-phase, and DNA index.

Tumor **grade** is frequently evaluated on the biopsy or surgical specimen and noted on the pathology report. Several grading systems for breast cancer exist, including the Nottingham and Bloom-Richardson scales. In general, low-grade tumors have less agressive features and are less likely to recur distantly, when compared to high-grade tumors.

Tumor markers are substances that can be detected in higher-than-normal amounts in the blood, urine or body tissues of some patients with cancer. Tumor marker tests that may be done on the breast cancer patient's blood include CEA and CA 27.29 (also called CA 15.3). These tests are usually only positive in bulky or advanced breast cancer disease, and therefore cannot be used for diagnosis or early detection. However, tumor markers may be used to follow the course of the disease, to determine the effect of treatment, and to check for recurrence. The usefulness of obtaining each test will be determined by the treating physicians.

Treatments

Many treatment methods are used for breast cancer. The treatment for an individual patient depends on:

- the type of cancer
- the size and location of the tumor in the breast
- the mammogram findings
- the results of lab tests done on cancer cells (including hormone receptors)

• the stage (or extent) of disease

• patient factors (health status, whether or not you have gone through menopause, treatment preferences, etc).

This list explains why two patients with seemingly similar diagnoses may receive different treatment recommendations. Treatment may also be influenced by further tests to determine whether the cancer has spread. A chest X-ray and blood tests to check the liver are standard in invasive disease. In more advanced stages, bone scans or CT scans of the lungs or liver may be indicated, since breast cancer tends to spread to these areas.

In **DCIS**, treatment is confined to the area of the breast and includes surgery with or without radiation therapy. Lymph node surgery and systemic (total body) drug and hormone treatments are not necessary because DCIS generally does not invade the lymphatic system or blood vessels to spread outside of the breast. The main goal is preventing a local recurrence in the breast or chest tissue. Some women with DCIS may benefit from taking medication that may reduce their risk of developing invasive breast cancer. Currently studies are evaluating tamoxifen and raloxifene for prevention of breast cancer. The role of these drugs should be discussed with an oncologist.

For **stages I and II** breast cancer, the initial treatment is usually surgery. If breast conservation (lumpectomy) is being done, surgery is usually followed by radiation therapy. Chemotherapy and/or hormone therapy are also usually recommended.

Treatment for **stage III** disease may start with either surgery or total body treatment (**neo-adjuvant** chemotherapy or sometimes hormone therapy), followed by surgery and possibly radiation.

Total body, or **systemic** treatment, given to patients with stages I, II, and III breast cancer, is aimed at reducing the likelihood of tumor spread in the future and at increasing the possibility of cure. This **adjuvant** treatment is supplemental to the local treatment with surgery and/or radiation therapy. It may include chemotherapy, hormone therapy, or both. Adjuvant treatment does not guarantee that distant spread of cancer will not occur in the future, but it does lower the likelihood.

A wide range of treatments exist for **stage IV** breast cancer, depending upon sites of spread, features of the tumor (such as hormone receptors), and the age, menopausal status, and general health of the patient. Stage IV breast cancer is generally viewed as an incurable disease, although there is wide variation in the number of years which patients may live with this disease, and there is optimism that some women may be cured with new forms of treatment.

Second Opinions

Most physicians will support a patient's efforts to obtain more information, including a second opinion, especially in making early decisions about breast cancer therapy. Many insurance companies will cover a second opinion regarding surgery. It may be advisable and helpful to include a radiation oncologist and a medical oncologist as consultants early in the treatment planning, in addition to a surgeon.

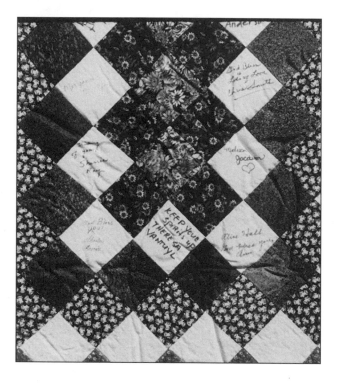

Friends of Anne Parker ❦ *An Act of Love* ❦ Quilt

7

Surgery for Breast Cancer: Mastectomy versus Lumpectomy, Axillary Lymph Node Dissection, Reconstruction

Breast Surgery

Surgery is the most common initial treatment for breast cancer. An operation to remove the breast is called a **mastectomy**. An operation to remove the cancer but not the breast is called **lumpectomy**, breast-sparing surgery, breast conservation, or local excision.

The goal in breast-sparing surgery is to remove the cancer surrounded by a rim of normal tissue, to obtain **clean margins**. Breast-sparing surgery is usually followed by radiation therapy to destroy any cancer cells that may remain in the breast and reduce the risk of cancer recurring.

In a total (or simple) mastectomy, the surgeon removes the entire breast and usually some lymph nodes from under the arm. In a modified radical mastecomy, the surgeon removes the breast, most of the lower and middle lymph nodes, the lining over the chest muscle, and sometimes part of the chest wall muscles.

For appropriately selected patients, there is no survival advantage for mastectomy when compared with breast conserving surgery and radiation. The 1990 National Institutes of Health (NIH) Consensus Conference on the Treatment of Early Stage Breast Cancer concluded that "breast conservation treatment is an appropriate method of primary therapy for the majority of women with stage I and II breast cancer and is preferable because it provides survival equivalent to mastectomy while preserving the breast."

The decision between a mastectomy and breast conservation depends on many factors, including:

- the patient's preference
- the size of the tumor
- the presence of DCIS, LCIS, **atypia** or **hyperplasia**
- the likelihood that all of the tumor can be removed without removing the entire breast
- the size of the breast
- the presence of **calcifications** on the mammogram
- the anticipated cosmetic result
- the ability to adequately monitor the patient for recurrences after surgery
- the patient's age and health
- a history of connective tissue disorders, like scleroderma
- the location of the nearest radiation facility
- previous treatment with radiation
- pregnancy (1st or 2nd trimester)

Some women who are not initially candidates for breast conservation may benefit from being treated with chemotherapy and/or radiation therapy before surgery. If the tumor shrinks significantly, they may then be able to have breast conservation surgery.

In most cases of invasive breast cancer, the surgeon also recommends evaluation of the lymph nodes under the arm (**axillary lymph node dissection or sentinel lymph node biopsy**) to help determine the stage of disease and plan further treatment. The standard axillary lymph node dissection removes all the lymphatic tissue below the large vein in the armpit area (level I and II nodes). Sentinel lymph node biopsy is a newer procedure that allows selected patients to have fewer lymph nodes removed. Sentinel node biopsy is currently being tested in clinical trials and these studies of its accuracy will ultimately determine whether it becomes part of the standard diagnostic procedures for breast cancer.

The sentinel lymph node is the first lymph node or nodes in the chain of nodes that drains the area of the cancer. They are identified by using a radioactive isotope marker substance and/or blue dye injected around the tumor. The marker and dye travel through the lymphatic channels and collect in the sentinel node(s). A special camera may be used to image the location of the sentinel lymph node preoperatively. During surgery the blue dye can be seen, and the lymph node radioactivity can be identified by a special hand-held isotope counter. Usually, pathologic analysis of the sentinel lymph node requires several days. If the sentinel lymph node has no cancer in it, no additional lymph nodes need to be removed. If there is cancer in the sentinel lymph node, then a full axillary lymph node dissection is generally recommended, due to a higher likelihood of additional positive nodes. If a sentinel lymph node cannot be identified during surgery, then the standard axillary lymph node dissection should be done.

Surgical Treatment Questions to Ask Your Surgeon

1. How much breast surgery do you perform in your practice?

2. Do I have a choice between breast conservation and mastectomy? Do you recommend one over the other for my particular circumstances? Why?

3. If I have a mastectomy and am interested in reconstruction, is it better to have it delayed or can I have it at the time of the mastectomy?

4. Am I a candidate for sentinel lymph node biopsy? What is your experience in doing this relatively new procedure?

Breast Reconstruction Surgery

Breast reconstruction is an option for a patient who has had a mastectomy. The decision to have reconstruction is an individual woman's choice. Many factors play into making this decision, and psychosocial support is available to help women with it. (See Psychosocial section.) Reconstruction may be started at the time of the mastectomy (**immediate reconstruction**) or may be done six months or longer after the mastectomy (**delayed reconstruction**).

Reconstruction typically involves either the insertion of an implant or a tissue transplant. **Breast implants** are plastic sacs filled with either silicone (a type of plastic liquid) or saline (salt water) which are surgically placed behind the chest muscle. Silicone implants are somewhat controversial and are not usually used.

In 1992 the U.S. Food and Drug Administration (FDA) declared a moratorium on silicon-filled implants — except for postmastectomy women in clinical studies — because of a lack of evidence supporting their safety. There have been reports of possible associations between silicone implants and connective tissue diseases such as scleroderma and lupus erythematosus. However, recently published studies do not clearly substantiate these associations.

Implants have been associated with the following risks:

- capsular contracture (hardening of the breast reconstruction because of scar tissue)
- leaking and/or rupturing
- calcium deposits in surrounding tissue
- shifting from the original placement site
- infection

Women considering breast implants should discuss these issues with their plastic surgeon and may want to contact the FDA for its most recent opinion on these devices.

Tissue transplants involve taking muscle, fat and skin from another part of the body and moving it to the chest area, where it is shaped into the form of a breast. These transplants are typically referred to as **flap procedures.** Tissue can be taken from either the lower stomach area (transverse rectus abdominus myocutaneous flap or **TRAM**), the back (latissimus dorsi muscle or LDM), or the buttocks (gluteus muscle). The TRAM flap is the one most commonly used for breast reconstruction. These are all major surgeries involving large wounds, significant recovery periods, and potential surgical complications such as poor wound healing and infections. Although there are definitely risks to these surgical procedures, many women report physical and emotional satisfaction from tissue flap breast reconstruction.

The choice of procedure may be limited by the patient's medical history, previous abdominal surgeries, body build, and smoking history. For a woman contemplating a mastectomy where reconstruction may be a consideration, a consultation with a plastic surgeon prior to mastectomy is advisable. Ask your breast surgeon for a referral to an experienced plastic surgeon or use a referral from the American Society of Plastic and Reconstructive Surgeons.

Breast reconstruction is a process that often takes several months to complete.

Frequently, surgery may be recommended on the other breast to make it more like the reconstructed breast. Washington State law requires health insurers to pay for reconstruction of the removed breast and/or surgery on the non-diseased breast to make it equal in size and contour. Medicare is required to pay for reconstruction. Medicaid will also pay if a case for medical necessity can be made.

There are information guides available that list questions to help you decide whether or not you want reconstructive surgery, what kind of reconstruction, and by whom. (See Reconstruction Questions below.) In addition, some surgeons have support and/or information exchange groups where women are encouraged to share information, observations and emotions. Inquire into these.

Reconstruction-Related Questions to Ask Your Surgeon

Selecting a Plastic Surgeon

1. How many breast reconstructions (implants and/or tissue transplants) have you done?

2. May I see pictures of your patients who have had reconstruction?

3. Can you put me in contact with someone who has had the procedure?

Understanding Reconstruction

1. What are the various types of reconstructive surgery?

2. What are the risks and potential side effects from each type? Will detection of a possible recurrence be difficult? Will there be pain? Will I need a special bra?

3. What can I expect the reconstruction to look and feel like? Will it be similar in look and feel to my healthy breast? Will there be differences over time — in three months, six months, a year? Will I have to have anything done to the healthy breast?

4. What type is best for me? Why?

5. When is the best time for me to have reconstruction— immediately after the mastectomy, or later, after chemotherapy and/or radiation therapy?

6. How many procedures will it take? How long will it take? Where will these procedures be performed? How much time will recovery take?

7. Will my insurance cover this type of surgery?

⊗RESOURCES

Selected articles, books and pamphlets

American Cancer Society. Breast Cancer Reconstruction after Mastectomy (1996) 800-ACS-2345

Berger, D., and Bostwick , J. A Woman's Decision: Breast Care, Treatment and Reconstruction (Third edition, Quality Medical Publishing, Inc., St. Louis, Mo., 1998) Revised and updated, a comprehensive resource about breast cancer surgical options and reconstructive surgery. Also includes interviews with survivors who discuss their results.

U.S. Food and Drug Administration. Breast Implants: An Information Update. Contains information about silicone gel-filled and saline-filled breast implants for reconstruction and augmentation. Covers issues such as FDA regulation, scientific studies, alternatives to breast implants and answers to frequently asked questions. For more information, call (888) 463-6332 or see the website at www.fda.gov/oca/breastimplants/bitac.html.

Bruning, N. Breast Implants; Everything You Need To Know (Hunting House, Alameda, CA, 1995) A valuable resource for any woman considering breast implants and for those who have them. Includes details of potential health risks, alternatives to implants, and advice on when and whether to remove them. A resource list is included.

American Cancer Society. Breast Reconstruction after Mastectomy (1996). Describes types of surgery with photographs and drawings, and gives answers to commonly-asked questions as well as a glossary of terms. 800-ACS-2345

See also Chapter 22: Breast Cancer Information. Some of the comprehensive books on breast cancer, such as Dr. Susan Love's Breast Book, contain thorough descriptions and discussion of reconstruction options.

Organizations

American Society of Plastic and Reconstructive Surgeons' Plastic Surgery Information Service, 444 East Algonquin Rd. Arlington Heights, IL, 60005. (800) 635-0635. Services: Information and referral for individuals seeking board-certified plastic surgeons.

Breast Implant Information Network, (800) 887-6828. Services: Directs women how to file complaints, and reports on the current status of various legal decisions.

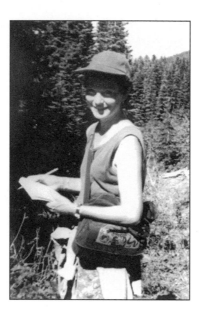

Shelly Minor

Diagnosed: Age 43, 1994

I fared my treatments well, but it was not without help. My friends and family poured out love and help, so I could concentrate on getting well. My devoted husband read me love poems, my son made me trays of tea, my daughter sang nonsensical songs to make me laugh. I do not remember that I had a disease as much as I had a job to do. I had to get well, I had a family to love, children to raise, a life to live. It was a gritting, frightening, soul-wearying time, and I learned that no kindness was too small. Every extended hand let us know that woven from all those hearts and hands was a saftety net of love and caring to support us.

8

Radiation Therapy

High-energy radiation can be used to kill cancer cells that may be present in the breast tissue. In most cases, a lumpectomy is followed by radiation therapy, to reduce the risk of local recurrence of the breast cancer within the remaining tissue. In some cases, radiation is also recommended following a mastectomy if there is a high risk of tumor cells remaining behind after surgery. This includes tumors extending to the edge of the surgery specimen, tumors close to the ribcage or chest wall muscles, very large tumors (greater than 5 cm), or tumors found in lymph nodes.

When radiation therapy follows breast surgery, a machine delivers radiation to the breast/chest wall and in some cases to the regional lymph nodes. The treatments are generally given five days a week for six to seven weeks. Each treatment takes a few minutes. At the end of the series, an extra **boost** of radiation is often given to the area where the cancer was found. During the actual radiation treatment, you will be alone in a room, but your radiation therapist will be able to hear and see you. You can't see or feel anything while the equipment is in operation; however, you can hear the machine being turned on and off.

A slightly longer initial radiation therapy visit, called a **simulation**, is required to determine the exact area to be radiated (called the radiation "port") and the set-up of the radiation machine. Tiny permanent skin tattoos or ink, and a cast or mold to keep the arm in the same position above the head, are generally used to assure that the radiation port is identical for each treatment.

Possible side effects of radiation include fatigue and skin irritation, such as itchiness, redness, soreness, peeling, or darkening of the breast. Other, more rare side effects of radiation in breast cancer patients can include radiation pneumonitis (inflammation of the lung tissue) or rib fractures. Radiation to the breast does not cause hair loss, vomiting, or diarrhea. Most side effects that arise during the course of radiation therapy will subside after the treatments have been completed. You are not radioactive during or after your therapy.

⊗RESOURCES

Books

Cukier D., M.D. Coping with Radiation Therapy (Lowell, 1994)

Dodd, M., R.N./Ph.D. Managing the Side Effects of Chemotherapy and Radiation (Prentice Hall, 1991)

Hunter, M., M.D. The Little Book of Breast Cancer (Cancer Info Press, 1998)

Lange, V., M.D. Be A Survivor: Your Guide to Breast Cancer Treatment (Lange Productions, 1998)

Publications:

National Cancer Institute. Radiation Therapy and You: A Guide to Self-Help During Treatment (Publication No.92-2227, 1993) Call (800) 422-6237, or fax request to (301) 330-7968.

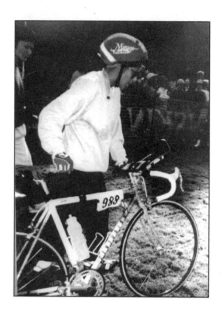

Kathleen Leonard
Diagnosed: Age 41, 1994

I wanted to be an example of how women can survive this kind of diagnosis and treatment and do it in a fashion that suits them. I also wanted to be a strong advocate for aggressive outreach/education and research in the cure for the disease, so I started a breast cancer support group in my community. I did so with the help of Team Survivor Northwest, the American Cancer Society, and the Tri-Cities Cancer Center. This group, "A Shoulder to Lean On," is now an example of how women afflicted with breast cancer are taking charge of their lives, SURVIVING, living life to the fullest, and bringing breast cancer awareness to others.

9

Chemotherapy and Hormone Therapy: Systemic Therapy, Implantable Catheters, High Dose/Stem Cell Transplants

༄

Systemic Therapy for Breast Cancer

In breast cancer, even when the tumor is small, cancer cells may have already spread beyond the breast. Surgery and radiation therapy are powerful ways of eradicating cancer within the breast and the adjacent lymph nodes. However, they are considered "local" therapies, because they have no effect on cancer cells that may have spread beyond the breast. Help in killing these distant cancer cells comes from chemotherapy and hormone therapy.

Therapies that circulate through the body's blood stream to attack cancer cells wherever they may have spread are called "systemic" treatments. Chemotherapy and hormone therapy given to breast cancer patients after their primary breast surgery are used to reduce the risk of later recurrence. These therapies are called **adjuvant therapies**. Chemotherapy given before breast surgery is called **neo-adjuvant** chemotherapy. If a patient's cancer has already shown signs of spread to distant sites (stage IV), then systemic therapy is generally used as the primary treatment.

Many breast cancer patients are cured by surgery (with or without radiation therapy) alone. Unfortunately, some patients develop recurrence of breast cancer in distant sites (including the liver, bones, and lungs). This can occur within months of the original diagnosis or many years later. Even the most sensitive blood tests and radiologic scans cannot detect these errant breast cancer cells at an early stage, when distant breast cancer is most curable. Since it is impossible to find small numbers of distant tumor cells with the techniques now available, recommendations about adjuvant therapy must be based on estimates of the chance that a patient's tumor cells have already spread through the blood stream or the lymphatic system to a distant site.

The decision about whether to include chemotherapy or hormone therapy in the breast cancer treatment plan weighs the possible benefits to be gained from the treatment with the risks and side effects of that treatment. The benefits could be a reduction in the likelihood of recurrence at a later time and a decrease in the chance of dying from breast cancer.

Many factors are taken into consideration when a treatment plan is being decided. The patient's age and menopausal status, the stage of the tumor (size, lymph node status, and evidence of distant spread), and the hormone receptor status of the tumor (estrogen and progesterone receptors) are considered. The pathologic grade of the tumor, DNA studies (ploidy, S-phase), and some oncogene studies (HER-2) may also influence the decision about whether or not a patient may benefit from systemic therapy.

Chemotherapy

Chemotherapy is the use of drugs to kill cancer cells and improve the cure rate. Chemotherapy may be given by mouth or by injection into a vein or muscle. The drugs then enter the bloodstream and travel through the body to attack cancer cells that may have spread from the original site. Adjuvant chemotherapy has been proven through large clinical trials to improve the cure rate and overall survival for breast cancer patients. Adjuvant chemotherapy may reduce the risk of recurrence in breast cancer by as much as 40 percent.

Chemotherapy for breast cancer is not all the same. There are different drugs, and also different recipes (or **regimens**) using combinations of drugs. Chemotherapy is given in cycles — a treatment period followed by a recovery period, then another treatment. Most current adjuvant breast cancer chemotherapy regimens include six cycles of treatment (usually over 6 months), although some regimens last four months and others can last for up to a year. The most common adjuvant breast cancer treatment regimens include combinations of one or more of the following drugs: doxorubicin (Adriamycin), methotrexate, 5-fluorouracil (5-FU), cyclophosphamide (Cytoxan), and paclitaxel (Taxol) or docetaxel (Taxotere). For patients with metastatic or recurrent disease, there are many other effective drugs as well, including trastuzumab (Herceptin), capecitabine (Xeloda) and vinorebine (Navelbine). Most patients undergoing chemotherapy for breast cancer are treated on an outpatient basis in a hospital or clinic. The nurses and pharmacists are specially trained and certified in cancer treatment.

All adjuvant chemotherapy regimens for breast cancer cause side effects, but most patients are able to do their usual activities most of the time (perhaps at a slower pace). Fatigue is the most common side effect, and often is worse near the end of treatment. Studies show that mild exercise can decrease the symptoms of fatigue. Many women treated for breast cancer experience some nausea. New, improved anti-nausea medications may be prescribed in those cases.

The blood cells that are made in the bone marrow (white blood cells that fight infection, red blood cells that carry oxygen, and platelets that help stop bleeding) can all be affected by the chemotherapy drugs. Levels of these blood cells are checked frequently while patients are receiving chemotherapy. Low levels of certain cells may lead to changes in chemotherapy doses, blood transfusions and/or the addition of blood cell growth factors. Growth factors are used to help boost the numbers of white cells (G-CSF or GM-CSF) or the red cells (erythropoetin).

Hair loss, skin and nail changes, changes in bowels, interruption of menstrual cycles, infections, and mouth sores (mucositis) are also potential side effects. Whether or not a certain symptom will occur depends both on the regimen and the patient. Your doctors and nurses are a good source of information on what to expect from the particular program that is being recommended. Most of the side effects from chemotherapy are short-term, and they will go away after completion of the treatment. Permanent side effects can include early menopause (permanent shut-down of the ovaries), rare cases of congestive heart failure from the drug doxorubicin (Adriamycin), and the even rarer development of pre-leukemia (myelodysplasia) and leukemia years after treatment.

Hormone Therapy

The growth of breast cancer cells, like the normal breast cells from which they are derived, can be affected by estrogen and other hormones. Hormone therapy for breast cancer may include the use of drugs to change the way that hormones or their receptors work. In pre-menopausal women, the use of surgery or drugs may be used to decrease hormone production by the ovaries. In general, hormone therapy is only effective if the breast cancer cells test positive for either the estrogen or progesterone receptor. These tests are a routine part of the work-up of a newly diagnosed breast cancer. Like chemotherapy, hormone therapy is a systemic treatment; it can affect cancer cells throughout the body.

Tamoxifen (Nolvadex), a drug that is taken by mouth, is the most common form of hormone therapy. It acts as an anti-estrogen, or a hormone blocker, on breast tissue and some breast cancers. Tamoxifen not only affects cancer cells, but it can also help prevent thinning of the bones (osteoporosis) and decrease the risk of heart attacks. Tamoxifen is an effective adjuvant treatment for breast cancer, and can also reduce the risk of recurrence by up to 40 percent. Evidence also suggests that tamoxifen can reduce the chance of developing a second breast cancer by up to 40 percent. Side effects include hot flashes, nausea, weight gain, and depression. Studies show that there is a slight increased risk of uterine (endometrial) cancer and blood clots for women on this drug, although these are quite rare.

Women taking tamoxifen should have an annual pelvic exam and notify their doctor of any unusual vaginal bleeding. The benefits of tamoxifen appear to be greater in post-menopausal women, and the side effects are worse in pre-menopausal women, which is why tamoxifen is most commonly used in older breast cancer patients.

Toremifene (Fareston) and raloxifene (Evista) are also anti-estrogens. Toremifene is recently FDA-approved for use in metastatic breast cancer. Raloxifene has been approved for prevention of osteoporosis, and is being investigated in breast cancer prevention.

Another class of hormone therapy, aromatose inhibitors, are effective for metastatic breast cancers and are being investigated in the adjuvant setting. Anastrozole (Arimidex) and letrozole (Femera) are newly approved aromatose inhibitors.

Bisphosphonates

Bisphosphonates are a class of drugs most commonly used to prevent and treat osteoporosis, since their main action is to prevent bone breakdown. Recent studies have shown that bisphosphonates added to chemotherapy or hormone therapy can reduce pain, fractures, and other complications of bone metastases due to breast cancer. Pamidronate (Aredia) is the bisphosponate most commonly used in the treatment of bone metastases. It is given as an intravenous infusion over 90-120 minutes every 3-4 weeks. New studies are investigating the use of bisphosphonates in the adjuvant setting, with the hope of preventing bone metastases from occurring.

Trastuzunab (Herceptin)

Trastuzumab is a new and innovative drug used to combat breast cancer which is over-expressing HER-2, which is found among 25 to 30 percent of women diagnosed with the disease. It is a monoclonal antibody, which targets the HER-2 receptor on the surface of the breast cancer cell. When a cell has too many HER-2 receptors, the cell is signaled to divide too often. The result is excessive growth of the cancer cells. Tumors that have excess HER-2 are called **HER-2 positive**; tumors that don't are called **HER-2 negative.**

Trastuzumab works by binding to the HER-2 receptors on the surface of the cell and suppressing excess growth. It has been studied in women with metastatic breast cancer and can be given alone or in combination with certain chemotherapy agents. It is given intravenously in an out-patient setting once a week and is generally well tolerated. The side effects can be fever and chills, mostly associated with the first dose.

Intravenous Access

Chemotherapy drugs can be introduced into the body in a number of ways, but most drugs are given intravenously (by vein). If the treatment is given by a needle into an arm (peripheral) vein, there are measures to take to make this a safe procedure. After breast surgery that involves lymph node dissection, it is important not to use the affected arm for intravenous infusion of chemotherapy drugs. The changes in circulation put a patient at a higher risk of infections and lymphedema in that arm. With some chemotherapy drugs it is important not to have blood drawn from the same arm that the nurses will use for chemotherapy. The nurses can use small needles to give the treatment, causing less irritation to the vein. Heat helps veins expand, making them easier to find. The source of heat can be a warm blanket or warm water from the faucet. Drinking lots of fluids will make the veins "plump" and easier to find.

For patients who are facing frequent chemotherapy treatments or longer infusions of chemotherapy, those who have hard-to-find or collapsible veins, or those who have a personal preference, there are catheters or shunts that can be surgically placed and remain in the patient for weeks or months. There are pros and cons to implantable venous catheters. The catheter eliminates the need to put needles into the arm for blood draws and chemotherapy. Placement of the catheter requires a surgery, although it is a minor outpatient procedure. If a definite recommendation of chemotherapy is made prior to the final breast surgery, the catheter device can be placed at the same time, eliminating the need for one more procedure. Placement of the catheter needs to be carefully determined to avoid irritation from clothing (like bra straps) rubbing on the site. Catheter complications can include infection, clots, or, rarely, a lung being punctured (pneumothorax) during the placement of the catheter. In general, they are very safe.

For some patients, a slow (continuous) infusion of a certain chemotherapy drug is part of the treatment regimen. In this case, some sort of implantable venous catheter is generally required. The patient can wear a pouch containing the drug in a "belt pack" with a pump. Some women wear their chemo pouch to work and the drug infuses slowly during the day.

Types of Implantable Venous Access Devices

All types of implantable venous access devices can be used to draw blood, infuse drugs, and transfuse blood. Your specific therapy may influence which type of device is best for you. Check with your medical team.

1. **Implantable Ports (Portacaths).** The port is a small disc about 1 1/2 inches in diameter. It has a raised center or septum which is made from a self-sealing rubber material. The septum is where the needle is inserted for delivery of medication or for blood draws. The medication is carried from the port into the blood stream through a small, flexible tube called a catheter. The port is inserted under the skin below the collarbone. Implantable ports can also be placed under the skin of the arm, above the elbow. Portacaths require a heparin (anti-clotting) flush every 3-4 weeks to keep the line flowing. They cause minimal alteration in appearance because they are totally under the skin, and there is no disruption to showering or bathing.

2. **External Sialastic Catheters (Hickmans, Broviacs, Groshongs).** An external catheter is a hollow tube made of rubber that is inserted into the large vein leading to the heart. The end of the catheter looks like an IV line in your chest. Blood draws and medication administration can be done directly from the end of the external catheter, avoiding needle sticks. The external catheters have a slightly higher rate of infections. These catheters require more home care, including daily heparin flushes and dressing changes. There is more of an alteration in body image and physical freedom with this type of catheter, due to the 4-5 inches of tubing extending from the chest wall. Care must be taken when showering, bathing and swimming.

High-Dose Therapy/Stem Cell Transplants

Although chemotherapy and hormone therapy can reduce the recurrence rate of breast cancer, and achieve remissions in patients with recurrent or metastatic breast cancer, they are not always successful. Oncologists are always searching for ways to improve the cure rate in breast cancer. In patients with stage IV (metastatic) disease, and earlier stage patients who are still considered to be at a very high risk of relapse following standard chemotherapy, "high-dose" chemotherapy regimens are being investigated in clinical trials as a way to improve the cure rate.

High-dose chemotherapy regimens use drug doses 5-10 times stronger than that given in standard adjuvant regimens, with the hope of overcoming the tumor's drug-resistance and achieving cure. The dose-limiting toxicity of many chemotherapy drugs is the effect on the bone marrow stem cells — the cells that give rise to the white blood cells, red blood cells, and platelets that circulate in our blood. Some high-dose regimens destroy the bone marrow (a process called myeloablation) as a side effect, and therefore require collection and reinfusion of a patient's own bone marrow stem cells. Other regimens do not require bone marrow stem cells, since they do not permanently eliminate all bone marrow cells. (These are "non-myeloablative.")

Formerly, the source of stem cells was a bone marrow harvest. This required anesthesia and a surgical procedure, in which needles were inserted in to the posterior pelvis/hip area to remove cells directly from the bone marrow. Today, the usual method of stem cell collection involves administration of growth factors (G-CSF or GM-CSF), and sometimes chemotherapy drugs, to stimulate the circulation of stem cells in the blood. These cells, which originate in the bone marrow, are called "peripheral blood stem cells." They are capable of repopulating the bone marrow after reinfusion. These cells are collected and separated from other blood cells by a process called "pheresis" using a special centrifuge. During the pheresis, the patient has two intravenous lines attached to the centrifuge: one line transfers blood from the body out to the centrifuge, and another returns blood from the centrifuge after the stem cells have been removed. The process takes 3-4 hours a day, and may require several days to collect enough cells. The cells are then frozen and stored until they are re-infused after the high dose therapy is given.

High-dose chemotherapy is usually given in the hospital over a period of several days. A central venous catheter is usually inserted before the treatment begins in order to facilitate the delivery of the chemotherapy, as well as the fluids, nausea

58   *Finding Your Way to Wellness*

medications, antibiotics, blood transfusions, and nutrition that are a typical part of the recovery process. If a stem cell re-infusion is part of the regimen, the stem cells are given after the completion of all of the chemotherapy. The blood cells made in the bone marrow (white blood cells, red blood cells, and platelets) drop to very low levels several days after the chemotherapy is given, and usually remain low for 10-14 days. During this time the patient will likely require antibiotics to reduce the chance of infection, as well as blood and platelet transfusions.

Side effects which are almost universal among all high-dose regimens include hair loss, mouth ulcers (frequently requiring narcotic pain medications), and nausea/vomiting. Many patients experience a decreased appetite that is often prolonged and may require the use of intravenous nutrition for a period of weeks. Other side effects are specific to the medications used in the regimen and may include damage to the lungs, liver, skin, and kidneys.

High-dose chemotherapy is sometimes recommended for stage IV breast cancer in remission, and to complete the adjuvant therapy of high-risk primary breast cancer (stage II or III, with 10 positive lymph nodes, or other high risk features). Early results of high-dose therapy in breast cancer patients were promising, and small non-randomized trials suggested that high-dose chemotherapy may indeed improve survival in selected breast cancer patients. Currently there is controversy about the benefits of high-dose therapy versus more conventional therapy. Results from large, well-planned clinical trials have yet to demonstrate their benefit to patients. High-dose therapy can be toxic, and patients undergoing this treatment should be treated as part of a clinical trial in an experienced center.

✍RESOURCES

Books

Mitchell, J. Winning the Chemo Battle (1991)

Burning, N. Coping with Chemotherapy (Dial Press, 1985)

Dodd, M., R.N/Ph.D. Managing the Side Effects of Chemotherapy and Radiation (Prentice, 1991)

Drum, D. Making the Chemothcrapy Decision (Lowell House, 1996)

McKay, J., R.N. Chemotherapy Survival Guide (New Harbinger, 1993)

Bazell, R. Her-2; The Making of Herceptin, a Revolutionary Treatment for Breast Cancer

Publications

National Cancer Institute. Chemotherapy and You: A Guide to Self Help During Treatment (Publication No. 94-1136, 1997) (800) 422-6237

National Cancer Institute. Research Report: Bone Marrow Transplantation and Peripheral Blood Stem Cell Transplantation (Publication No. 95-1178, 1994) (800) 422-6237

National Cancer Institute. The Immune System: How It Works (Publication No. 92-3229) (800) 422-6237

Internet

Genentech BioOncology, HER-2 and Trastuzumab (Herceptin) website: www.her2.com

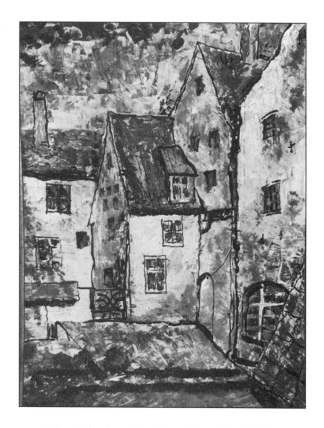

Irina Kalendarev ❧ *Narrow Street* ❧ Painting

10

Management of Side Effects:
Nausea, Head Coverings, Prostheses, Lymphedema

Coping with the side effects of treatment can be both physically and emotionally challenging. Having psychosocial support from the very beginning may make meeting the challenges easier. Surgery raises issues related to prostheses, bras and/or reconstructive surgery. Side effects from chemotherapy and/or radiation often bring hair loss and skin changes. Fatigue drains patients' energy for coping with all the changes.

Nausea, Pain, Eating Problems

It is important for new patients to know that today we have much better ways to manage these side effects than we did even a few years ago. The important thing is that you feel comfortable working with your medical caregivers as a team. This means that you inform them of any changes that you experience, so that together with you they can manage your care most effectively. Managing nausea or pain sometimes takes several attempts before the best results are obtained. This means you must not give up if the first prescription brings disappointing results. Let your caregivers know so they can try other medications or protocols. A relatively new class of anti-nausea drugs is called "serotonin uptake inhibitors." Drugs in this class tend to cause less sedation and other side effects. Ondansetron (Zofran) and ganistetron (Kytril) are two of these agents. Both are available as intravenous injections and in pill form. If eating becomes a problem, nutritionists with experience helping other cancer patients are available. Ask for a consult.

Fatigue

Many patients say that fatigue is the most bothersome side effect of treatment. It is hard not to have your usual energy, not to be able to do even basic tasks sometimes. It is important that you let your caregivers know when you are tired and how tired you are — so that medications and transfusions can be given if appropriate. Erythropoetin (Epogen, Procrit) is a growth stimulator for red blood cells that can help to boost the blood count and decrease anemia. Often, however, you will have to manage your fatigue by making some adjustments in your routine. Prioritize your tasks and make sure you are doing the most important tasks when you still have energy. Learn to say "no." Learn to accept help that may be offered from family and friends, or ask for the help you need if it is not offered. Eat foods high in nutritional value to the extent you can. Maintain some exercise program if at all possible. When women don't feel well, they often stop exercising altogether. Research is showing, however, that maintaining some level of mild exercise (walking, swimming, yoga) may actually increase energy levels in people undergoing cancer treatments. We are also finding that taking only very short naps during the day improves quality of sleep at night and also helps improve energy levels.

Skin Changes

Various changes in skin texture and color can be expected when one is undergoing radiation and/or chemotherapy. All inflammations, blisters and rashes should be brought to the attention of your physician as soon as possible. Following good personal hygiene during treatment, especially brushing your teeth, is important. Most conditions fall into the category of dry skin and changes in skin pigmentation. During treatment, alcohol-based products, harsh clothing (e.g., wool), sun exposure, hot baths, and certain preparations (e.g., deodorants) may contribute to skin problems. It is probably best to avoid these. Over-the-counter moisturizers and sunscreens have been found to be helpful. Protective clothing with properties similar to topical sunscreen preparations is also now available. (See retailers at the end of this chapter.) The National Cancer Institute (NCI) has booklets which provide advice on what to expect and what to do.

Hair Loss

The loss of hair, or alopecia, has its own challenges. Developing strategies prior to losing your hair from treatment works best for many women. This often involves getting a short haircut in order to reduce the shock of hair loss. Special attention should also be paid to your scalp and hair during treatment, using mild shampoos and hairbrushes.

The choice of whether or not to wear a wig or other head covering, is an individual one. Numerous retailers have various products available. The American Cancer Society (ACS) provides a list of local retailers. In addition, various videos and pamphlets provide instructions on how to tie and make head wraps. (See resources.) If a friend offers to help, suggest that he/she buy you a nice cotton scarf for a head wrap. Women have also found night caps especially helpful for providing comfort and warmth.

Here are some tips for getting a wig that looks and feels good:

- Be measured for a wig only after you have lost your hair — sizes change without hair.

- Avoid obtaining a wig in a box from a mail order retailer— it is difficult to get one which is comfortable and looks good.

- Select an experienced retailer— ideally a licensed cosmetologist, so she can clip or shave your head and fit and style the wig as well. Select a retailer who is available and convenient for you. (See resources.)

Some people have found borrowing a wig from their hospital and/or local ACS patient services department helpful. Insurance policies may, or may not, cover a wig with prescriptions from your physician. Talk with retailers regarding financing options prior to purchasing.

Cosmetic needs may also change. Many women discuss their needs with their cosmetic salespeople and have found them quite helpful. Some retailers have designed special programs to help women determine their cosmetic needs, identify products and learn application techniques (e.g., how to create the illusion of eyelashes and brows when you don't have any). The National Cosmetology Association has also prepared a special pamphlet, "Look Good...Feel Better," and works with ACS Patient Services to offer free cosmetic consultations through a joint program also called "Look Good...Feel Better."

ⓥRESOURCES: Skin Care and Head Coverings

Selected articles, books and pamphlets

Noyes, D. ,and Mellody, P. Beauty and Cancer: A Women's Guide to Looking Great While Experiencing the Side Effects of Cancer Therapy (1992)

National Cancer Insitute. Chemotherapy and You (publication No. 94-1136, 1996) 800-4-CANCER

National Cosmetology Association's CTFA Foundation. Look Good...Feel Better: Caring for Yourself Inside and Out (1995) 800-4-CANCER

American Cancer Society. Making Your Own Headwraps Even If You Don't Sew! (1992) (800) 227-2345

National Cancer Insitute. Radiation and You (1999) 800-4-CANCER

American Cancer Society. Resource Guide for Cancer Patients Experiencing Hair Loss (1994) (800) 227-2345

Coping: Living with Cancer (a magazine), 2019 N. Carothers, Franklin, TN 37064. (615) 790-2400. Contains articles on beauty and skin care. Many doctors' offices and treatment facilities have copies.

Organizations

American Cancer Society (ACS)
(800) 227-2345
Services: Provides assistance with obtaining wigs. Works with the National Cosmetology Association to offer the "Look Good...Feel Better" cosmetic consultation program. Provides pamphlets on how to make and tie headwraps.

Beauty and Cancer Program
Volunteer Services
University of Washington Medical Center
(206) 598-4218
Services: personal consultations on head coverings and skin care. Free cosmetic samples, wig bank.

National Cosmetology Association
CTFA Foundation
800-395-LOOK
www.cancer.org
Services: Provides a pamphlet with cosmetology tips, and works with ACS
to provide consultations.

National Cancer Institute (NCI)
800-4-CANCER (800-426-6237)
Services: Provides a nationwide telephone Cancer Information Service
(CIS). Answers questions and forwards fact sheets and booklets.

Sun Precautions
(800) 882-7860, or (206) 322-7057
4015 Madison, Seattle, WA 98112
Services: Provides head-to-toe sun protection clothing and some
sunscreen products.

Y-ME
(800) 221-2141
Services: Provides prostheses for a nominal mailing fee.

Retailers

"Tender Loving Care," ACS, 1996 (a mail order catalog with head
coverings, hair pieces and prostheses which may be ordered at reduced
prices)

Look through the yellow pages in the local telephone books under "wigs
and hairpieces." Many retailers provide catalogues and pamphlets on their
products and how to use them. Ask for copies. Some retailers (e.g.,
Nordstrom) provide complimentary makeup applications by professional
makeup artists who have received training in the special needs of cancer
patients. Special makeup techniques and products are often suggested.

Prostheses and Bras

One of the issues after breast cancer surgery is selecting an appropriate prosthesis. Mastectomy patients generally are instructed not to wear a bra for several weeks after surgery, until their incision is adequately healed and swelling has subsided. Your physician will be able to determine when you are physically ready to proceed with a consultation at a prosthesis retailer. It is recommended that you obtain a postoperative garment to use after surgery if you are more comfortable in a supportive undergarment and will be proceeding with working or social functions. The choices available in this category are:

Softee: a cotton camisole garment that fits snugly against the body with no inside seams to irritate incisions. Prices on these items vary depending on the manufacturer and are available where breast prostheses are sold. The size range is xs-xxlg to accommodate a variety of body types; the wearer adds fiberfill into pockets as needed to achieve a normal shape. Softees may be reimbursed by your insurance provider but usually require a physician's prescription. In the case of Medicare reimbursement, the prescription must be dated AFTER the date of surgery. Some hospitals routinely provide these items in their post-surgery care.

Leisure Bra. Longer elastic banding under the bustline area and cotton fabric make these a comfortable choice to transition into a more traditional style bra. Front hooks allow easy access for dressing without straining the underarm area. This type of garment can be a good choice during radiation. Contour shaping can be added with a foam or prosthesis form or fiberfill stuffing. Sizing is generalized: 34-46 A/B, C/D.

Not every woman who has a mastectomy chooses to wear a breast prosthesis or breast form. The decision to wear, or not wear, one is a matter of choice. A breast prosthesis may assist women in adapting to changes in body appearance and weight distribution after a mastectomy. They are made from silicone, foam or fiberfill. Some prostheses fit into a bra with or without special pockets holding them in place. There are also several prosthesis options that attach to the body. One system involves special adhesive strips that apply to the chest wall, and the breast form attaches with a Velcro inset. The second choice is a breast prosthesis with a silicone gel strip that enables it to attach directly to the chest wall without strips. Many women enjoy the freedom of movement that an attachable form introduces, since the weight is on the front of the body instead of on the shoulder area.

Prostheses come in various shapes, sizes and colors to accommodate different body types, breast shapes, surgeries and personal preferences. Getting a good fit is important, and it may require fortitude and patience. Some women report that taking along an experienced friend (or a Reach to Recovery volunteer) is helpful. Finding an experienced retailer is also important. The prosthesis should match the remaining breast in order to maintain body weight equilibrium and prevent back, neck and posture problems. Also communicate to your fit consultant your lifestyle activities so she can help you select a form that is appropriate for you. Schedule at least an hour for your initial fitting appointment so you have enough time to make a comfortable decision without being rushed. Many women also investigate prosthesis options prior to their surgery so they can make educated choices about their options after surgery.

Many surgeries involve only partial breast removal, or lumpectomies and breast conserving methods. There are a number of options available to help with symmetry after these types of surgery. Check with a certified fitter to investigate preferred bra styles that equalize the size and shape of breasts, or partial silicone shells that add slight contouring but not the weight of a full form.

After breast surgery it is important for a woman to be fitted for a comfortable and supportive bra. Make sure the bra fits and supports you, hugging the chest wall and the underside of the arm and cup area. No flesh should overflow the top or underarm area. If you have an existing breast, make sure the bra fit contains the full breast capacity; then the prothesis form can be sized appropriately for the other side. The bottom of the bra should fit so that it anchors down comfortably snug, low on the small of the back (not over the shoulder blades). The front of the band should fit flush against the chest wall so the center tacks and there is no gaping or bowing at the top. Straps should not cut into the shoulder since the bra should be supporting from under the bustline — not pulling from the top. For bra fit after a bilateral mastectomy, try a style with a fuller band on the bottom to help anchor the bra down, and fuller coverage on the top edge so the forms don't fall away from the body when you bend over.

Since many retailers will modify bras for use with prostheses free or at a nominal charge, bring with you to the fit appointment the style of bra you were wearing prior to surgery if you are happy with the fit. It is important to note that prosthesis products will vary in price according to the quality, warranty and comfort.

Most insurance providers will cover the cost of breast prostheses and mastectomy bras, especially if the physician writes a prescription with medical necessity documentation. It is important to verify individual eligibility and coverage with your insurance group before purchasing these products. It is also wise to bring a prescription or referral for all items being claimed to your insurance provider to your fitting. Medicare does cover a percentage of the cost of products, but the prescription should be dated before the date of purchase. Many retailers are familiar with insurance requirements and may be able to help facilitate the process.

Women without insurance have options, as well. They may contact their local American Cancer Society patient services or Y-ME for assistance with securing a prosthesis free or at a nominal charge.

⊗RESOURCES: Prostheses

Organizations

American Cancer Society
(800) 227-2345
Services: Provides information, referrals to Reach for Recovery Volunteers, and assists with obtaining prostheses for low-income women.

Y-ME
(800) 221-2141
Services: Provides information and prosthesis bank. Will send a prosthesis anywhere, if appropriate size is available, for a nominal fee.

Protheses Resources, cont.

NATIONAL RETAILERS WITH 800 NUMBERS

Bosom Buddy
(800) 262-2789
Products: prostheses.

Camp Heathcare, Inc.
(800) 492-1088
Products: prostheses, fiberfill forms, lingerie and swimwear.

Coloplast
(800) 726-6362
Products: Discrene-self supporting breast prosthesis. Products are listed within the Medicare price range. Brochure and video available.

Freeman
(800) 253-2091
Products: prostheses and bras.

JC Penny, Inc.
(800) 222-6161 (24-hour order line)
Products: prostheses and bras. Medicare may be billed under some circumstances.

Jodee, Inc.
(800) 423-9038
Products: prostheses, bras and accessories.

Spenco
(800) 877-3626
Products: prostheses, bras and accessories

Y-ME
(800) 221-2141
Services: prostheses for a nominal mailing fee.

LOCAL RETAILERS

• *Bremerton:*

Cuvertino's Intimate Apparel
(360) 373-3140
810 6th, Bremerton
and
15952 Levin Rd N.W.
Poulsbo, WA 98370
(360) 779-5216

Farrell's Home Health
(360) 377-0164, Or 800-233-6265
2325 Wheaton Way
Bremerton, WA 98310

Medequip Services, Inc.
(360) 479-8811, or 800-542-5775
2329 Wheaton Way
Bremerton, WA 98310

• *Edmonds/Everett:*

Cornerstone Prosthetics and Orthotics, Inc.
(425) 339-2559
1300 44th St.
Everett, WA 98203

Nova Care Hanger Prosthetics Orthotics, Inc.
(425) 353-5385
206 E. Casino Rd., Suite 5
Everett, WA 98208

LOCAL RETAILERS, continued

Knudson Herb Surgical Appliance and Hospital Equipment
(425) 259-0144
2909 Hewitt Ave.
Everett, WA 98201

• *Olympia/ Centralia:*

Novacare/Hanger and Orthotics
(360) 459-1099
208 Lilly Rd. NE
Olympia, WA 98506

• *Seattle Area:*

Greater Seattle Prosthetic & Orthotic Center Inc.
Numerous locations; see yellow pages

Mary Catherine's
(206) 322-1128
901 Broadway
Seattle, WA 98122
and
(206) 783-7030
2232 NW Market
Seattle (Ballard), WA 98105

Nordstrom
Downtown Seattle
(206) 628-2111, ext. 1240
Bellevue Square
(425) 455-5800, ext. 1240
Northgate
(206) 364-8800, ext. 1240
Southcenter

(Nordstom continued)
(206) 246-0400, ext. 1240
Alderwood Mall
(425) 771-5755, ext. 1240
Tacoma Mall
(253) 475-3630, ext. 1240

Northwest Prosthetic and Orthotic Clinic
(206) 323-4040
600 Broadway
Seattle, WA 98122

Healthtech Medical
(206) 621-0290, 800-426-1634
1213 Madison
Seattle, WA 98104

• *Tacoma/ Puyallup:*

Judy's Intimate Apparel
(253) 474-4404
4538 S. Pine
Tacoma, WA 98407

Linda's Post Mastectomy Boutique
(360) 897-8398
21505 145th St. E.
Sumner, WA 98390

Lymphedema

Lymphedema is an abnormal accumulation of lymphatic fluid (water and protein) in the soft tissues of the body. It is usually due to obstruction of the lympatic ducts. In breast cancer patients, lymphedema can occur in the arm, hand, and/or chest wall on the side of the body that had surgery. Factors which contribute to the onset of lymphedema include axillary node dissection and/or radiation therapy. Removal of lymph nodes causes a decreased rate of flow of the lymphatic fluid as it passes through the remaining nodes. Radiation to the chest wall and armpit causes scarring in the lymph vessels, which also slows down the rate of flow of the lymph system in this region. This allows lymph fluid to accumulate within the vessels and tissue spaces.

Over time, the fluid accumulates to the point that the skin is actually stretched. This may be the first symptom of lymphedema. Other early symptoms include: heaviness, weakness, tingling, numbness, achiness, decreased flexibility in your hand or wrist, and pain anywhere in the affected arm. Some women do not experience any symptoms, while others have severe complaints. Initially, the swelling will fluctuate with activity. Many people believe that since the swelling goes away with rest, they don't need treatment. However, this is exactly when treatment should be started. If caught in the very early stages treatment is less time consuming and results are obtained much more quickly.

Lymphedema may occur at any time following breast cancer treatment. Some women develop symptoms within the first year and others 20 years later. Infections involving the affected extremity may also trigger the onset of lymphedema. The risk of developing lymphedema after breast surgery or radiation varies widely, depending on the type of treatment and the patient's body. Only a small percentage of breast cancer patients develop severe lymphedema, but many women experience mild symptoms, especially following significant arm activity.

Ask your surgeon to explain lymphedema and its treatments to you before surgery. Some doctors recommend seeing a physical therapist before or immediately after surgery to learn ways to prevent lymphedema and other post-surgery problems. Regaining full motion and strength of the arm and shoulder blade following treatment, along with the prevention of infection, are the best options for decreasing the risk of developing lymphedema.

You will need to take special care of the affected arm for the rest of your life, so learn how to prevent injuries and infections and what to do should one occur.

Some things to be aware of are as follows:

- Avoid any type of trauma to the affected arm (bruising, cuts, sunburn or other burns, sports injuries, insect bites, cat scratches).

- Use an electric razor rather than a safety razor to avoid nicks.

- Try to avoid injections or blood draws in the affected arm. Have blood pressure checked in the unaffected arm. (Note: it may be necessary to have blood drawn from this arm during chemotherapy, so that the drugs can be injected in the unaffected arm.)

- Avoid heavy lifting with the affected arm.

- Avoid vigorous, repetitive movements against resistance with the affected arm.

- Do not wear tight jewelry or elastic bands around affected fingers or arms.

- Avoid cutting cuticles when manicuring hands.

- Keep your weight down. Avoid tobacco, alcohol, and salt.

Lymphedema is best treated when caught early, so call your doctor at the first sign of swelling or infection. If the lymphedema is caused by infection, your doctor will prescribe appropriate antibiotics. (Some women carry a prescription with them when they travel.) If the lymphedema is not caused by infection, a treatment plan will be determined using methods that could include manual lymphatic drainage, bandaging, compression garments, and exercises.

Physical therapists, occupational therapists and massage therapists treat lymphedema. Most patients are referred to these specialists by surgeons or oncologists. As long as you have physical therapy/occupational therapy benefits or rehabilitation benefits as part of your insurance coverage, and a licensed physical/occupational therapist provides the treatment, the services will be covered. Problems arise when individuals have policies that limit the monies allowed for physical/occupational therapy treatment.

㊈RESOURCES: Lymphedema

National Lymphedema Network
2211 Post Street, Suite 404
San Francisco, CA 94115
(800) 541-3259
www.lymphnet.org
This nonprofit resource center provides patients and professionals with information about prevention and treatment. Services include a hotline for referrals for medical treatment and physical therapy, general information and support in your area. An information packet is available.

Northwest Lymphedema Center
1800 NW Market, Suite 203
Seattle, WA 98107-3908
(206) 782-5598
This local nonprofit sponsors a support group, a newsletter, and workshops. It is dedicated to "providing education, information and resource referral to those interested in, or suffering from, lymphatic system disorders."

Breast Cancer Physical Therapy Center
1905 Spruce Street
Philadelphia, PA 19103
(215) 772-0160
This organization specializes in women with breast cancer, helping them deal with range-of-motion problems and lymphedema. It publishes a booklet, Recovery in Motion, and has helped set up numerous breast rehabilitation centers throughout the U.S.

Books

Stumm, D. Recovering from Breast Surgery: Exercises to Strengthen Your Body and Relieve Pain (Hunter House, 1995)

Love, S., and Lindsey, K. Dr. Susan Love's Breast Book (Addison-Wesley, 1995)

Foldi, M., M.D .and Foldi, E. M.D. Lymphedema: Methods of Treatment and Control (Lymphedema Association of Victoria, 50 St. Georges Rd. Upper Beaconsfield, Victoria 3808, Australia)

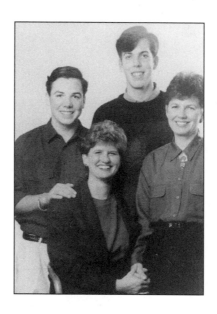

Desiray Bailey, M.D.

Diagnosed: Age 45

Throughout my breast cancer experience, I have been blessed with the people in my life. My life partner has been the most loving, supportive partner a person could hope for. I continue to experience an abundance of love and support from my family and my friends. My colleagues and co-workers were considerate and gentle in their administrations. My support group has been an ongoing source of support and care. I only hope I can give back at least some of what I have been given.

11

Clinical Trials

ஐ

What is a clinical trial?

Advances in medicine and science are the direct result of new ideas and approaches developed through careful research. In the field of medicine, research studies conducted with patients are called clinical trials. A clinical trial is an organized study which tries to answer specific scientific questions and to find new and better ways to prevent, diagnose and treat diseases. Participation in clinical trials could potentially benefit many people by providing treatments in addition to what currently exist, and by increasing knowledge about a disease and its potential treatments. Clinical trials are an extremely important way to evaluate new approaches to diseases, such as cancer, and a scientific way to test new agents or procedures while ensuring safety.

What types of clinical trials exist?

There are many kinds of clinical trials. They range from studies of ways to prevent, detect, diagnose, control and treat cancer to studies of the psychological impact and ways to improve the patient's quality of life and comfort. In cancer research, a clinical trial generally refers to the evaluation of treatment methods such as a new drug or a new way of using known standard drugs and treatments. Cancer clinical trials that deal with new approaches to treatment most often involve the use of surgery, radiation therapy, hormone therapy, and/or chemotherapy, alone or in combination. A new area of cancer treatment is biological therapy, which uses substances which affect the body's own ability to fight the disease. Depending on what is being studied, a particular trial may involve patients with cancer or people who do not have cancer but are at higher risk than most people for developing it. Many of today's most effective interventions are the direct result of knowledge gained through clinical trials.

The search for good cancer treatments often begins with basic research in the laboratory and in animal studies before they are tested in patients. Based on what researchers learn from laboratory studies, as well as from previous clinical studies, new therapies are designed to take advantage of what has worked in the past and to improve on these techniques.

What is a protocol?

A protocol is a carefully constructed treatment plan investigating an experimental procedure or treatment. It is designed to answer research questions and to protect the patient. The protocol explains what the trial will do, how and why. An investigator is an experienced clinical researcher who prepares the protocol and uses it in the treatment of patients.

Who can participate in a trial?

In order to most accurately evaluate the effectiveness of a treatment, clinical trials must be carefully managed and follow strict scientific guidelines. Eligibility criteria are specific characteristics that are used to identify people who can participate in a certain trial. In most cancer treatment trials, results will only be reliable if everyone has certain specified, similar aspects of their disease. Some other common eligibility requirements are: age, general health, the stage and extent of disease, previous treatments, and the type of cancer. These criteria also help ensure the safety of participants by protecting them from known risks.

Where are trials conducted?

In the U.S., clinical trials may be conducted or overseen by the National Cancer Institute (NCI), a cooperative group (an organized group of oncologists from a number of hospitals and clinics), or an institution (a qualified oncologist or group of oncologists in one institution or clinic.) Most clinical trials are conducted at major academic medical centers, but patients can also receive their treatment at a local medical center or physician's office, depending on the type of trial. Community hospitals and doctors are becoming a significant part of the research network. Community Clinical Oncology Programs (CCOPs) link community physicians with National Cancer Institute clinical research programs, so that more cancer patients can participate in clinical trials in their own community.

Major cooperative groups involved in breast cancer clinical trials are the National Surgical Adjuvant Breast and Bowel Project (NSABP), the Southwest Oncology Group (SWOG), the Cancer and Leukemia Group B (CALGB), and the Eastern Cooperative Oncology Group (ECOG.) In the Pacific Northwest, the Puget Sound Oncology Consortium (PSOC) coordinates many clinical cancer trials.

What are the phases of clinical trials?

Clinical studies are conducted in steps called phases, each designed to find out certain information. Patients may be eligible for studies in different phases, depending on their general condition and the type and stage of their cancer. Each new phase of a clinical trial depends on and builds on information from an earlier phase.

Phase I cancer studies determine the safety of a new treatment. In a Phase I study, a new research treatment is given to a small number of patients. These treatments have been tested in laboratory and animal studies but not in humans. Phase I studies of new drugs determine how best to give the drug (orally, intravenously, etc.), how often, and how much can be given safely. Although the research treatment has been well tested in laboratory and animal studies, the side effects in patients cannot be completely known ahead of time. Since Phase I studies may involve significant risks and are of unproven benefit, they are generally not offered to patients who have other, proven treatment options available to them. Phase I studies may produce anticancer effects, and some patients have been helped by these treatments.

These studies often involve dose escalation, by starting with a low dose not expected to cause serious toxicity in any patients, and then increasing the dose for subsequent patients according to a preplanned series of steps. The dose can be increased by giving more at one time or by giving the same dose more often. Once the best dose is chosen, the drug is studied for its ability to shrink tumors in Phase II trials.

Phase II cancer studies determine the effect of a research treatment on cancer and are designed to find out if the treatment actually kills cancer cells in people, and also to generate more information about the safety and risks. Phase II studies are conducted with larger numbers of patients and usually focus on a particular type of cancer.

Phase III cancer studies are designed to determine whether a new treatment is more effective and/or less toxic than a standard therapy. If a treatment shows activity against cancer in a Phase II study, it moves on to Phase III. In Phase III studies, the new treatment is directly compared to the standard one (the treatment most accepted), to see which is more effective.

Large cooperative group studies are important because it typically requires many patients to determine whether two treatments are actually different, or whether the difference could be due to chance. Statistical results are influenced greatly by the number of patients treated in the study, with larger studies having a greater likelihood of obtaining a definitive answer about treatment differences.

How are patients protected?

One of the ways to prevent the bias of a patient or doctor from influencing study results is randomization. A randomized clinical trial is a Phase III study in which patients with similar traits (such as extent of disease) are assigned by chance to one of the treatments being studied — either the new intervention or the standard intervention. Because irrelevant factors or preferences do not influence the distribution of patients, the treatment groups can be considered comparable and results of the different treatments used in different groups can be compared.

The group that receives standard (or the most commonly accepted) treatment is called the control arm and receives what experts view as the best treatment available. The group receiving the experimental therapy is called the experimental arm and receives a treatment that experts think may have equal benefit or advantages over the standard treatment. Sometimes no standard treatment exists for certain groups of patients. In drug studies for such cases, one group of patients might receive the new drug and the other group none. No patient is placed in a control group without treatment if there is any known treatment that would benefit the patient. Patients in the control group are monitored as often and as carefully as those in the treatment group.

A double-blind study is one in which neither the patient nor the physician knows which drug (or dose) the patient is getting. In single-blind studies, patients do not know which of several treatments they are receiving — to prevent personal bias from influencing a patient's reactions and study results — but the medical team does. In blinded studies, the treatment can be quickly identified, if necessary, by a special code.

To further prevent the bias of the medical team or the patient from influencing study results, placebos and other blinding procedures are sometimes used. A placebo is an inactive substance resembling a medication, used as a control to compare a medicine believed to be active. It is usually a tablet, capsule or injection that contains a harmless substance but in appearance is the same as the medicine being tested. A placebo may be compared with a new drug when no one knows whether any drug or treatment will be effective.

An Investigational New Drug (IND) is a drug allowed by the Food and Drug Administration (FDA) to be used in clinical trials but is not approved for commercial marketing or general use. New cancer treatments must prove to be safe and effective in scientific studies before they can be made widely available. Phase IV is a term sometimes used to describe the continuing evaluation of a new drug as it is used after FDA approval and in combination with other treatments.

With any new treatment, there may be risks as well as possible benefits. Today, clinical trials are regulated by a number of governing groups and processes to ensure patient safety and comfort, and benefit from scientific research. Patients' well-being during clinical trials is most notably protected by the informed consent process, peer review, and an Institutional Review Board (IRB) that scrutinizes all research involving humans.

The process in which a patient learns about the purpose and protocol of a clinical trial and agrees to participate is called **informed consent**. Anyone entering a clinical trial is required to sign a form indicating that she understands what will and may happen during the study. It is crucial that an individual receive and clearly understand as much information as possible before agreeing to participate in a clinical trial. Patients must be aware of the treatment to be given, medical procedures, side effects and the possible risks and benefits. Patients should decide whether they want to take part in a study only after they understand both the possible risks and the benefits. The informed consent also indicates which costs are covered by the study, and states clearly that patients have the right to leave the study at any time without giving up access to other treatments. This decision, along with any questions concerning the study, should always be discussed between the patient and her health care team.

Does insurance cover the cost of clinical trials?

Although clinical studies are an integral part of cancer treatment, some insurance policies do not reimburse patients' costs for clinical trials or experimental drugs. Fortunately, the majority of insurance companies recognize that patients enrolled in cancer clinical trials would require therapy whether or not they are in a trial, and do cover most of the medical costs for such patients. The National Cancer Institute provides some limited treatment in Bethesda, Maryland, without charge to patients enrolled in an NCI study.

In trials involving investigational new drugs, patients are sometimes provided with free drugs or procedures, although they are charged for clinic costs. Cancer center financial counselors and clinical research study coordinators should be able to help patients determine and obtain insurance coverage for a given study. A doctor's letter that outlines the study protocol and documents the patient's eligibility for the trial may sometimes be necessary to obtain insurance company approval for a clinical trial.

Why do patients participate in clinical trials?

Patients take part in clinical trials for many reasons. Usually, they hope for benefit for themselves. They hope for a cure of disease, a longer time to live, or a way to feel better. Often they want to contribute to a research effort that may help others. Knowledge gained from clinical trials has been essential to progress in understanding breast cancer, and these studies continue to play a key role. Major scientific discoveries in the laboratory are leading to exciting new approaches against breast cancer. The goal is to translate the best of that research into findings that directly help patients. Clinical trials, the link between basic research and patient care, offer hope for the future.

℘RESOURCES

Publications

National Cancer Institute. What Are Clinical Trials All About? (NCI Publication No. 92-2706, 1992, (800) 422-6237)

National Cancer Institute. Patient to Patient: Cancer Clinical Trials and You (Video, (800) 422-6237). Limited to one video per person.

National Cancer Institute. Taking Part in Clinical Trials: What Cancer Patients Need to Know (NCI's new, easy to understand brochure designed for cancer patients and their families. Call the NCI's Information Services at (800) 422-6237 to request a free copy, or download it from the Cancer Trials web site: http://CancerTrials.nci.nih.gov)

Internet

DOD Tricare Breast Disease Clinical Trials Page
Compiled by Walter Reed Army Medical Center
http://breastd2.wramc.amedd.army.mil
The National Cancer Institute and the Department of Defense have an inter agency agreement providing TRICARE/CHAMPUS-eligible patients access to NCI-sponsored clinical trials throughout the country.

National Cancer Institute's Clinical Trials Page
http://cancernet.nci.nih.gov/trials
Up-to-date information on over 1,500 ongoing cancer treatment trials.

NABCO (National Alliance of Breast Cancer Organizations)
Homepage, Trials News section: www.nabco.org
Brief descriptive summaries of 150 breast cancer trials are available in lay language, along with a search capacity.

National Library of Medicine's Clinical Trials Page
www.clinicaltrials.gov
This site includes listings of trials sponsored by pharaceutical companies as well as those that are government- and university-sponsored.

Other Services

National Cancer Institute's Cancer Information Service
800-4-CANCER [(800) 422-6237]
For information about clinical trials being conducted in your area. Services are provided in English and Spanish.

National Cancer Institute's Cancer Fax
(301) 402-5874
Information about cancer sent by fax machine. (Use the handset of the fax machine to respond to instructions and activate the faxing of the information requested.)

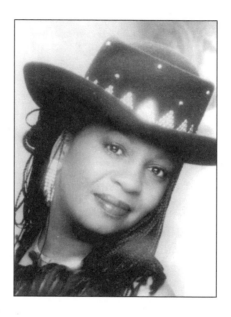

Bridgette Richardson

Diagnosed: Age 35, 1996

It has been very important for me throughout my experience to talk
with friends and family who offered their encouragement. In particular,
one of the things that I did to stay positive was to sing, "His Eye Is on
the Sparrow." Now, I try to encourage other people to take charge of
THEIR life by being more knowledgeable about their own health.

12

Incorporating Complementary Therapies into the Treatment Program

𝔊ᴥ

Overview

Complementary Therapies (CTs) are those treatments and strategies that are used in addition to "conventional" medicine. They include nutritional supplements; herbs; diets; lifestyle changes; massage; manipulation of joints; exercise; mind-body strategies including visualization, imagery, meditation and hypnosis; acupuncture and oriental medicine; and more. Some of these treatments offer benefits such as cancer preventive actions, enhanced immune system functioning, improved quality of life and solutions to some specific health issues. Although CTs can contribute significant benefit to the overall cancer treatment program for a patient, they are not intended to replace proven, "conventional" anti-cancer treatments. CTs should be used with care, since they have the potential to interfere with chemotherapy, radiation, and surgery. In addition, they can actually worsen side effects when used inappropriately.

CTs have enjoyed a great increase in popularity as well as health claims. The most common kinds of therapies and providers are listed below. If you have an interest in a CT that is not described here or simply want to evaluate these more closely, you will likely benefit from the services of a licensed provider.

Kinds of Complementary Therapies

Diet and Nutrition

Diet and nutrition can play a positive role in cancer prevention as well as your general health. Many of the diet and nutritional supplements are reasonable, while others are extreme. If you plan to revise your diet and improve your nutrition, it can be helpful to enlist the support of a licensed health care provider.

Acupuncture and Oriental Medicine

Needles and Chinese herbs are used in a system of diagnosis with logic and applications that often differ significantly from Western thinking. Acupuncture and Oriental medicine have been used to treat many different human diseases in Asia. Acupuncture has been shown to be useful for the control of nausea and vomiting as well as some painful conditions.

Botanical (herbal) medicines

Botanicals offer a wide variety of treatment actions. Many modern drugs are based on herbals. Some of the herbs that are available over the counter have actions in your body as strong as some prescription drugs. Homeopathy is a unique version of botanical medicine.

Herbals can, in some cases, provide safe effective treatment for a wide range of ailments. They can also, however, interact with drugs or other conventional treatments and may have side effects that are not well explained on the label.

The best results are usually achieved by doing your homework and enlisting the help of an expert. Consult with your licensed providers if you are also receiving conventional treatment, in order to avoid an unexpected interaction.

Massage Therapy

Massage therapy has been well accepted by many cancer survivors. A few simple precautions and checking in with your physician will give you a safe, rewarding entry to this comforting therapy.

Music Therapy

Music therapy, like counseling, can provide benefits of relaxation and comfort.

Counseling

Counseling can provide relaxation, stress relief and perspective during difficult times. In some cases, counseling can help you reduce stress and increase your coping skills with just a few visits. It is important to find a counselor whose interests, experience and perspective mesh well with yours.

Manipulation

Manipulation of the spine and extremities can sometimes provide pain relief and improved function. There are significant variations in the services available from different licensed providers. Find one who shares your objectives. Check with your oncologist or other provider to be certain that there are no exceptional circumstances to be considered.

Physical therapeutics, including exercise

Physical therapeutics can reduce pain and improve function for a wide variety of complaints. When exercise is part of the program, there can be an added disease prevention component.

Sources for Complementary Therapies

There are a number of sources for CT treatment, including naturopathic physicians, acupuncturists, massage therapists, chiropractors, physical therapists, counselors and more. Some have specific training and knowledge for dealing with the special considerations of cancer survivors. The most commonly utilized provider types are described below.

Naturopathic Physicians

In Washington State naturopathic physicians are licensed primary care providers who utilize clinical nutrition, botanical medicine (herbs), some Chinese medicines, manipulation, counseling, massage, some physical therapy, and other natural therapies. In addition, naturopathic physicians can write prescriptions for certain drugs and perform some office surgery procedures. Most specialize in certain areas and some offer additional services such as hydrotherapy, acupuncture and natural childbirth.

Naturopathic physicians strongly support the body's innate ability to heal itself but also cooperate with conventional medical interventions. Naturopathic physicians utilize the designation N.D., which is not the same as M.D.

Acupuncturists and Oriental Medicine

In Washington State, acupuncturists are licensed by the State of Washington Department of Health. They practice Traditional Chinese Medicine (TCM), which can include acupuncture, traditional Chinese herbs, heat therapy (moxibustion), massage, exercises and dietary advice. The objective of Chinese medicine is to help the body heal.

TCM is considered by some to be a type of energy medicine, focusing and treating the body's energy in "meridians" that traverse the body. Acupuncturists utilize the designation LAc, which is not the same as M.D.

Physical Therapists

Physical therapists are licensed by the State of Washington to provide a wide variety of treatments ranging from exercises to therapeutic heat, light and sound. These treatments can be useful for regaining full function following treatment, as well as for helping specific problems such as lymphedema. Physical therapy is often but not always provided on a referral basis from your primary health care provider.

Licensed Massage Practitioners

In Washington State, massage practitioners are licensed. They provide an array of different kinds of massage protocols. Massage therapy can provide important relaxation and other suggested benefits for cancer survivors. Many massage therapists do not treat cancer survivors because of concerns about harming the patient, but this modality can be utilized safely and effectively when coordinated with your primary provider.

Counselors

Licensed counselors can provide a variety of services, including stress counseling, imagery, visualization, and other mind-body strategies.

Other Sources for Complementary Therapies

Some categories of CT providers are not licensed or regulated by the State of Washington. These include music therapists, some exercise trainers and others. If you are pursuing these directions, it is usually best to find a referral from someone you trust, such as the staff of an existing provider. Other support organizations such as Cancer Lifeline can also provide helpful information.

Considerations for Getting the Best Result

There are many unregulated sources of information about CTs, including the internet, salespersons and significant media coverage. Some of this information is accurate and some is not.

CT treatments are available from licensed providers and unlicensed practitioners, and some can be purchased over the counter. While State licensure and other regulatory functions help protect the public from untrained and unethical providers, such protections do not exist with unlicensed persons. "Certifications" by organizations that are not government regulated may not be meaningful. There are numerous claims made on the internet and by salespersons. Some are accurate and others are inaccurate.

When using CTs, it is important to be certain that you are getting quality advice that is specific and correct for your particular circumstance. The following guidelines will help you:

• Utilize services from providers licensed by the State of Washington Department of Health. Unlicensed providers can be anyone walking on the street with minimal or no training.

• Insist that your medical specialists know about all treatments that you are pursuing.

• Require that all treatment-specific providers such as naturopathic physicians, acupuncturists etc., provide your medical specialists with written reports of what they are doing.

• Ask for referrals. Medical specialists and staff are often a good source for finding CT providers who understand the special needs of cancer survivors.

☺RESOURCES

Organizations

Professional Licensing Division
State of Washington Department of Health
1300 SE Quince St.
Olympia WA 98504
Phone: (360) 236-4501 or (360) 236-4800
(For regulated providers)

Cancer Lifeline
6533 Fremont Ave. N.
Seattle, WA 98103-558
(206) 297-2100; 24-hour lifeline: (206) 297-2500 or (800) 255-5505
www.cancerlifeline.org
Offers free services for cancer patients and caregivers, including
relaxation and visualization series, nutrition classes, 24-hour lifeline,
family support programs, kid's group, exercise workshop and yoga.

Wellness Works
Evergreen Community Healthcare
12040 N.E. 128th St., Suite 120
Kirkland, WA 98034
(425) 899-2264
email: jjones@echc.org
Offers information and support for those with cancer and chronic health
challenges.

Books & Publications

Chopra, D. Ageless Body, Timeless Mind (Harmony, 1993)

Chopra, D. Quantum Healing: Exploring the Frontiers of Mind/Body Medicine (Bantam, 1989)

Ellis, A., Wiseman N., Boss K. Fundamentals of Chinese Acupuncture (Paradigm 1991)

Goenka, S. Vipassana Meditation (Harper Collins, 1987)

Goldberg, Definitive Guide to Cancer (Future Publishing, 1997)

Kaptchuk, The Web That Has No Weaver (Dongdon and Week, 1983)

Kornfield, J. A Path With Heart (Bantam, 1993)

Labriola, D. Complementary Cancer Therapies (Prima, 1999)

Moyers, B. Healing and the Mind (Doubleday, 1993)

Novak, J. How to Meditate (Crystal Clarity Publications, 1989)

Pizzorno, J. Total Wellness (Prima, 1996)

Rose, J. The Aroma Therapy Book: Applications and Inhalations (North Atlantic Books, 1992)

Seigel, B. Love, Medicine and Miracles (Harper Collins, 1988)

Susan G. Komen Breast Cancer Foundation. Facts for Life: Alternative and Complementary Therapy (800) 462-9273

PRR Publications. In Touch (Periodical for patients describing new advances and other issues in cancer treatment. (516) 777-3800)

Meditations in Radiation
by Jan Slawson

The dolphins surround me
   they reassure me
   they sing and they touch me

The waves wash the cells away
   and break them into tiny bits of sand
      to be absorbed
      by my body

Blue water, grey dolphins,
   healing, purging the blackness
   of the cancer

My father's hand outstretched
   the light from God
   through his fingers
   into my breast
   to heal
   and to give life, a second time

Invisible rays
Burning a pattern in my chest
Killing the unwantedness
Leaving a scar of memory

The End

A kiss goodbye from the sea of calmness
The dolphins bid me farewell
The death funnels out like pieces of sand
   Through the pores — It's over!

A new beginning

13

Using Exercise and Nutrition in the Fight Against Breast Cancer

ॐ

Nutrition

A growing body of research supports the effect of diet on health. Obesity, low intake of fruits and vegetables, high fat diets, and high alcohol intake have all been implicated in increasing the risk of developing breast cancer. There may also be a link between these dietary factors, particularly being overweight, and a higher risk of breast cancer recurrence. Excess fat stores can raise the levels of certain hormones in the blood that can promote the growth of breast cancer cells. Some researchers have suggested that monounsaturated fats, which are present in high amounts in olive oil and canola oils, may lower a woman's risk of breast cancer.

There is evidence that breast cancer is less common in countries where the typical diet is high in soy. Isoflavones, which are sometimes called phytoestrogens or plant estrogens, are found in soy foods. They have properties similar to human estrogen, but are much weaker. Isoflavones have beneficial health effects, including decreasing symptoms associated with menopause such as hot flashes, and decreasing heart disease and osteoporosis.

Studies looking at dietary intake of soy and the risk of breast cancer suggest that isoflavones may have a protective effect against breast cancer. Laboratory studies have shown conflicting data, with breast cancer stimulation or inhibition depending on which cell lines, type of isoflavone, and dose of these agents are used. Phytoestrogens can be very helpful in managing menopausal symptoms in breast cancer survivors. However, some doctors feel that women with estrogen-receptor positive breast cancer or those who are on tamoxifen should minimize their intake of isoflavones until we have a better understanding of the effect of phytoestrogens on breast tumors.

Some researchers have focused on fruits and vegetables, and their contents of vitamins and minerals, as links between diet and breast cancer risk. Vitamins contain substances called antioxidants, which work to repair the cell's DNA after it has been damaged by a number of causes, including X-rays, sunlight and chemicals. Some vitamins, such as the vitamin A-related retinoids and B-carotene, can regulate the growth of cancer cells. There are clinical trials underway testing the effects of some of these vitamins in breast cancer patients.

Breast cancer survivors have a higher than average risk of developing a second breast cancer, in addition to their risk of a recurrence of the original breast cancer. Nutrition and diet are factors over which women can take control following a breast cancer diagnosis. Good general recommendations for a healthy diet that may reduce the risk of developing breast cancer or prevent its recurrence include:

- Take off excess weight

- Minimize the amount of red meat, saturated fat, salt, and sugar

- Eat a balanced diet with a good variety of nutrients and plenty of fiber (fruits and vegetables)

- Any alcohol intake should be in moderation

Resources

Dietitians can best be located through the health care facility where you are receiving your care. It is important to differentiate between dietitians who have graduated from accredited schools and are registered to practice, and nutritionists who may not be credentialed.

National Cancer Institute. Eating Hints for Cancer Patients (NIH Pub. No 94-2079) (800) 422-6237

Keim, R., and Smith, G. What to Eat Now: The Cancer Lifeline Cookbook (Sasquatch Books, 1996)

Simone, C. Cancer and Nutrition (Avery Publication Group, Inc., 1992)

Exercise

Energy levels during cancer treatment and recovery after surgery will be different for every person, depending on the extent of the disease, the treatment received, and other factors. Exercising after surgery will help regain motion and strength in the arm and shoulder. Exercises can begin slowly and gently shortly after surgery, and gradually become more active. Exercise is encouraged during radiation therapy and chemotherapy.

Regular gentle exercise may help combat fatigue and enhance well-being. It also helps with weight control. A study recently published in the *Journal of the National Cancer Institute* indicates that "moderate", regular physical activity may reduce a woman's risk of developing premenopausal breast cancer by up to 60 percent.

Many patients feel they would benefit from an exercise program during or after treatment, but are unsure about what would be best for them and how to start. Ask your physician for a referral to the physical therapy program at your clinic or hospital. A physical therapist can teach you specific exercises to strengthen the major muscle groups of the legs and arms, as well as stomach exercises to help regain the strength needed to perform your daily routine. This will also help fight fatigue.

There are also community-based groups to help breast cancer patients exercise. They are listed below. Remember, these are group classes and provide general information.

Cancer Lifeline Movement Awareness Workshops

To assist women of all ages who have experienced cancer in regaining personal power and control through the use of movement, dance and exercise. (206) 297-2100 or www.cancerlifeline.org

Team Survivor Northwest

Team Survivor Northwest is a project initiated by women cancer survivors of all ages. This dedicated group is committed to giving survivors the support, skills, and knowledge needed to achieve their fitness goals.

Team Survivor Northwest promotes fitness through regularly scheduled exercising and training sessions. This education and support allow women to participate in local walking, running, swimming and cycling events at all ability levels. Other activities include hiking, snow-shoeing, and cross-country skiing. (206) 732-8350 or www.teamsurvivor.org

Yoga

Many individuals find yoga to be beneficial physically, mentally, and spiritually. Check your local Yellow Pages, or ask others who practice yoga about various centers. Refer to the section on Spirituality.

Qi Gong

Qi Gong is an active and intrinsic physical exercise which regulates the mind, breath, and body. Regular practice can build one's mental consciousness, strengthen internal functions, and bring into balance both the body and mind.

Qi Gong can be classified as "hard" or "gentle" gong. The "hard" belongs to martial art; the "gentle" refers to health preservation, or "Qi Gong Therapy." Qi Gong can also be divided into "moving" (moving externally and calm internally) and "calm" (calm externally and moving internally).

Tai Chi

Tai Chi consists of movement and exercise routines designed to balance the energies within the body as well as the mind. It is similar to, yet different from, Qi Gong.

For more information

Qi Gong Association of America
27133 Forest Springs Lane
Corvallis, OR 97330
(541) 752-6599

John Bastyr University
14500 Juanita Drive N.E.
Bothell, WA 98021
(425) 823-1300
Contact this university's library for information.

Wellness Works
Evergreen Hospital
12303 N.E. 130th Lane
Kirkland, WA 98034
(425) 899-2264

Northwest Institute of Acupuncture and Oriental Medicine
701 N. 34th, Suite 300
Seattle, WA 98103
(206) 633-5581

Oregon College of Oriental Medicine
10525 S.E. Cherry Blossom Drive
Portland, OR 97216
(503) 253-3443

Taoist Studies Institute
225 N. 70th
Seattle, WA 98103
(206) 784-5632

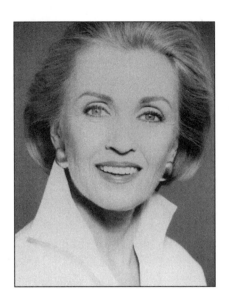

Jan Slawson
Diagnosed: 1991 and 1993

After my diagnosis, I wanted to assist other women through their breast cancer with support and health education. I accomplished this by chairing the first annual Komen Race for the Cure® in Seattle in June 1994. Afterward, I served two years as secretary to the board of directors of The Puget Sound Affiliate of the Susan G. Komen Breast Cancer Foundation. I have been president for the past two years.

14

Follow-up Care and Survivorship

ॐ

Follow-up Care

Completing cancer treatment means having mastered a new language, finished various therapies and managed any side effects that may have arisen. Regular follow-up exams continue after breast cancer treatment and are important. These checkups usually include exams of the chest and breasts, underarm and neck. Annual Mammograms, pap smears, and gynecologic exams are also part of follow-up care.

There are several tests that are not normally considered standard follow-up procedures for breast cancer. However, it is important that women be aware of them. While there is not enough evidence that the majority of women will benefit from them, these tests are helpful for some women. These tests include complete blood counts, bone scans, ultrasounds of the liver, and breast cancer tumor marker tests.

Having had cancer in one breast gives you a higher-than-average risk of developing cancer in the other breast. Breast self-examination, checking both the treated area and the other breast, should be done monthly.

Tell your doctor about other physical problems if they occur: pain, loss of appetite, changes in menstrual periods, skin reddening or thickening, or nipple discharge. Most symptoms do not turn out to be related to breast cancer, and your doctor can reassure you about them.

Survivorship

All patients look forward to finishing their treatments; however, it is not unusual for patients to find their feelings changing as the last treatment appointment approaches. For many people, treatment means fighting their cancer. Even though they understand the treatment has accomplished its purpose, they feel that if they stop, they will be vulnerable to cancer's return.

Treatment time can be so occupied with medical appointments, work and families, that emotions surface only when treatment is completed. It is useful to talk about these feelings with others — your physician and nurse, other patients, your family. Some people find that their efforts to live a healthy lifestyle help them to feel that they are still doing something to help themselves to remain cancer-free.

Other patients find that they actually miss the routine of treatments, and miss the contact and support they got from staff and other patients. Patients can find it hard to lose regular contact with others who understand the cancer experience and what they have been through.

You, and those around you, may expect life to return to "normal," but life is not the same as before your diagnosis. You may still be experiencing fatigue or other side effects for some time after ending treatment. You may find it difficult to do the work you used to do. You may find your illness affects employment or your insurance. If you do experience problems, remember you are not alone. Thousands of other patients have gone before you, and their experiences can help you handle concerns that arise. Many support groups welcome women who have completed their treatment. Creating a place for cancer in your life but keeping cancer in its place is a task of survivorship.

ⓈRESOURCES

Books

Benjamin, H.H. From Victim to Victor: The Wellness Community Guide to Fighting for Recovery for Cancer Patients and Their Families (Jeremy P. Tarcher, Inc., 1985)

Halvorson-Boyd, G., and Hunter L. Dancing in Limbo: Making Sense of Life after Cancer (Jossey-Bass, 1995)

Harpham, W. After Cancer: a Guide to Your New Life (Norton, 1994)

Hoffman, B. A Cancer Survivor's Almanac (Chronimed Publishing, 1995)

Johnson, J., and Klein, L. <u>I Can Cope: Staying Healthy with Cancer</u> (DCI, 1988)

Mullan and Hoffman, editors. <u>Charting the Journey: An Almanac of Practical Resources for Cancer Survivors</u> (Consumers Union, 1990)

Nessim, S., and Ellis, J. <u>Cancervive</u> (Houghton Mifflin, 1991)

Weiss, M.C., and Weiss, E. <u>Living Beyond Breast Cancer</u> (Times Books, 1997)

Publications and Products

National Cancer Institute. <u>Facing Forward: A Guide for Cancer Survivors</u> (National Cancer Institute Pub. No. 94-2424) (800) 422-6237

National Coalition for Cancer Survivorship (Selected audio cassettes) Toll Free: (888) 650-9127, (817) 866-5748 for cassettes.

Organizations

National Coalition for Cancer Survivorship
1010 Wayne Ave., 5th Floor
Silver Spring, MD 20910
Toll Free: (888) 650-9127

The Wellness Community
2716 Ocean Park Blvd.
Santa Monica, CA 90405
(888) 793-9355

Threads of Life (A knitting support group for cancer survivors)
Tanya Parieaux
Seattle, WA
(206) 938-9081
email: tanypar@aol.com

Wellness Works
Evergreen Healthcare
12303 N.E. 130th Lane, Suite 120
Kirkland, WA 98034
(425) 899-2264
email: jjones@echc.org

Offers "Living with Intention" program

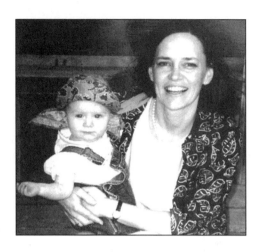

Mary Clarfeld
Diagnosed: Age 33

My greatest joy is my family. I dearly love my son, who is married to a wonderful woman. I have four terrific stepchildren, a great husband, and a beautiful new daughter! Having a baby after breast cancer was something I never thought possible, and I have been two feet off the ground since she was born. I feel very lucky to have had so much happiness, and I am looking forward to many years of joy.

15

Recurrence: Dealing with Mortality

☙

Before the widespread use of adjuvant systemic treatment, about 50 percent of breast cancer patients who had a cancer recurrence were found to have distant spread of their cancer within three years after diagnosis, and 90 percent in five years. Five years was therefore viewed as a landmark, or a point at which patients could be declared "cured." With more and more patients being diagnosed at earlier stages, and more women receiving adjuvant chemotheraphy and hormone therapy, an overall decrease in the number of breast cancer recurrences is being achieved. In addition, there may be a shift toward later detection of recurrences. While a woman who has had breast cancer can never be 100 percent certain that she is cured forever, the likelihood of future recurrence still decreases with time elapsed from the initial diagnosis.

All patients hope that, once treatment is completed, their illness will never return. If it does, it is a shock. Many patients say it is more frightening and difficult than the original diagnosis. Initially, it is a common fear that recurrence means a death sentence, but the courses of metastatic breast disease are diverse, variable, and largely unpredictable. Knowing this can be frustrating when making long-range plans, yet this knowledge is also a source of hope. Many women are living with advanced disease for a number of years, often well beyond statistical medical predictions. Some see their illness as a chronic condition which allows for new meanings and shifting priorities. Living fully, in the face of uncertainty, becomes the focus.

Cancer recurrence can be a time for individuals to examine philosophical and spiritual issues that we all should consider, but often avoid or postpone. It is not unusual for patients who have been forced to face these issues to talk about how important and valuable the process was for them. People often say, "I sure didn't want my cancer, but my life is so much better now than before because of the ways my experience has changed my outlook." They note how their priorities have changed and how this has freed them from many unnecessary concerns.

People come to this emotional resolution in different ways. Some have a spiritual base that can help them deal with issues such as the meaning of their life and their mortality. Others find answers in literature or by talking to friends, family members, or a counselor. This can also be a time when the understanding of others in similar circumstances, as in a support group, can be of great help. Discussing disease and death-related concerns within one's closest relationships can be a difficult and delicate process, but in a group of empathic peers, there is freedom of expression and sharing. It seems that what is important is for people to be able to identify what matters to them most, what gives hope or meaning to their life, and what is their own personal truth.

Hospice

Hospice services are designed to provide support for people in the last phase of terminal illness. The term "hospice" originally was used to describe a place of shelter and rest for ill or fatigued travelers on long journeys. Hospice focuses on "palliative" treatment, relieving symptoms and improving quality of life, as opposed to "curative" treatment. It seeks to provide a pain-free, dignified life in patients' homes, hospitals and other health care settings.

Hospice services are provided by a team of caregivers who work with the patient's physician and may include a nurse, social worker, home health aide, physical or occupational therapist and/or volunteer. Medical services, emotional support, spiritual and other counseling, and practical services are offered. Hospices help support family and friends in providing day-to-day patient care at home. Services are covered by Medicare, Medicaid and many private insurance companies. Hospice care can be arranged by contacting your physician or health care facility.

Ⓢ RESOURCES

Books

Colgrove, M. ,Bloomfield, H.H., and McWilliams, P. How to Survive the Loss of a Love (Bantam Books, 1977)

Grollman, E. Talking about Death; Dialogue between Parent and Child (Beacon Press, 1976)

Grollman, E. Straight Talk about Death for Teenagers: How to Cope with Losing Someone You Love (Beacon Press, 1976)

Krauss, P., and Goldfischer, M. Why Me? Coping with Grief, Loss and Change (Bantam Books, 1990)

Mayer, M. Advanced Breast Cancer: A Guide to Living with Metastatic Disease (O'Reilly Assoc., 1998)

Middlebrook, C. Seeing the Crab: A Memoir of Dying (Basic Books, 1996)

Stein, S. About Dying: An Open Family Book for Parents and Children Together (Walker, 1976)

Pamphlets

Coping; Living With Cancer (a magazine), 2019 N. Carothers, Franklin, TN 37064, (615) 790-2400

National Cancer Institute. Advanced Cancer: Living Each Day (NCI Publication No. 93-856) (800) 422-6237

National Cancer Institute. Patient Guide; Managing Cancer Pain (NCI Publication No. P476) (800) 422-6237

National Cancer Institute. Questions and Answers about Pain Control: A Guide for People with Cancer and Their Families (NCI Publication No. P122) (800) 422-6237

National Cancer Institute. When Cancer Recurs: Meeting the Challenge Again (NCI Publication No. 93-2709) (800) 422-6237

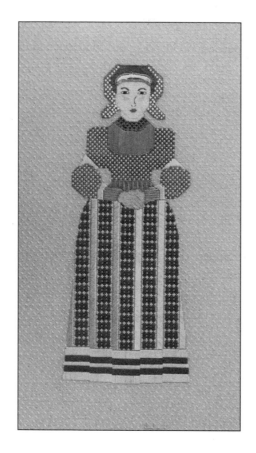

Lillian Hofflan ✌ *Anne of Cleve* ✌ Needlepoint

16

The Psychological Impact of Breast Cancer: Emotions, Personal Relationships, Sexuality, and Support Groups

❦

Emotions

It is not unusual for patients to feel anxiety or depression as they deal with so many changes and so much uncertainty. This is not a sign of weakness, but a normal reaction to an extraordinary situation which has overwhelmed a person's resources. It is important to let your medical caregivers know if you feel that depression or anxiety is interfering in your life. Often these feelings are a signal that you may not have allowed yourself sufficient time or opportunities to express your feelings. Or you may need more assistance and support to meet your needs. Talking with a counselor a few times often can give patients an opportunity to identify troubling feelings that need to be expressed, to receive reassurance that their feelings and reactions to their illness and treatments are very normal, and to find more support. Talking with someone whom you feel really understands can provide much relief.

Antidepressant medications have been found to be helpful by many patients during this difficult time. Patients sometimes resist taking "yet another medication," and others feel that admitting to the need for an antidepressant represents a weakness or a failure. However, these medications can be a valuable tool to help women manage their feelings more effectively. Women have reported that the medications gave them a way of evening out their emotions and finding the energy to cope more effectively with their situation.

Family and Children

For some women, a great concern is how their illness will affect their children. The tendency is to try to protect children by withholding information. This usually does not work well — children are extremely sensitive and pick up family concerns. They may seem disinterested, but they overhear conversations and phone calls, and are alerted by changes in their normal schedule. What helps children to cope best is to be told the truth in a way appropriate to their age level, and to trust that they will be kept informed. Children are amazingly resilient and can tolerate tough situations if they feel included in events, are told what they can do to help, are reassured that they in no way caused the problem, are reassured about how their schedule will continue, and are told who will be available to take care of them if a parent is unavailable. It helps children to meet your doctor, to see where you go for treatments, and to know that they can help by playing quietly or by drawing you a picture. Some books to help you with your children's concerns are listed in the resource section.

Questions about how to talk about your illness may come up with your spouse or partner as well. Again, talking as openly and honestly as possible works best. Sometimes it is easiest for you to initiate this by saying something like, "We have been focused on me and my illness; how is all this for you? What has been hardest for you? What is scariest?" Hearing their concerns may open communication by letting them know you recognize that they are affected by your illness as well. Cancer impacts the whole family, and managing it works best if the family copes together. Sometimes it helps to think of the family as a "team." Coping takes "teamwork."

Because each family member has special roles, you need to keep your signals straight by having regular team meetings to check how the game is going and to prepare for the next scrimmage. Often what is hard for family members is seeing you suffer and feeling helpless to do anything meaningful to make things better for you. You can help them best by letting them know realistic ways they can support you. One of the things most women find very supportive is for their partner or another close person to really listen to them. You may find it helps to tell the person how useful that is, and to let him or her know that you need someone to listen and understand as you sort out your feelings. They need to know that if they can do this, they will be giving you a valuable gift. Your knowing they understand and care can give you the strength to handle difficult situations.

Caregiving by Family and Friends

Changing routines. The impact of breast cancer is felt by the whole family. Most hospitals have social workers available to support and counsel the patient and family. Other family members need to share the workload, but the patient should be encouraged to continue to do as much as possible. Friends of the family may also be asked to provide support and assistance.

More than flowers and a get-well card. There are many ways family and friends can help a breast cancer patient undergoing treatment:

- Stay in touch, send a funny card, or visit.
- Encourage others to stay in touch.
- Listen to and respect your loved one's feelings.
- Prepare meals and encourage others to do the same. Let the patient know who will be bringing meals and on which days.
- Offer to do household chores.
- Offer to run errands for the patient.
- Offer to take the patient to doctor visits.
- Treat the patient with respect.
- Organize a care team.
- Water the plants.
- Do the laundry.
- Do the grocery shopping.

Taking care of the caregiver. Caregivers and family members can become overwhelmed and need to take care of themselves as well as the patient. They need to determine their abilities and limits, and then make genuine offers of assistance that are not undue sacrifices. Assess the situation and involve others to assist with the caregiving when you have reached your limits.

Body Image and Sexuality

Breast cancer patients may experience several types of body changes: changes in or loss of the breast due to surgery, lymphedema (swelling) of the arm after node dissection, loss of hair due to chemotherapy, and changes in sexual functioning due to dryness caused by chemotherapy or menopausal symptoms (like hot flashes) that may also be brought on by the chemotherapy. It is crucial that you are informed about any of these changes that you may experience. This gives you the opportunity to adjust to them, to find out what you can do about them, and to work through your feelings about them. The goal is for you to feel proud of your ability to tolerate your treatments and not feel any loss of self-esteem because of the changes in your body. This is not always easy. Talking with other women with breast cancer, either alone or in a support group, can help. The book, *Spinning Straw into Gold*, by Ronnie Kaye, has a good discussion about adjusting to a new body image. A counselor can also help women to grapple with these very personal feelings and maintain self-esteem. If you have a partner or spouse, it is very important that there be open sharing about these issues.

A key issue with partners is dealing with body changes, especially changes in or the loss of your breast. Many women feel they are unacceptable after surgery, and imagine that their spouse feels the same way. If they cannot talk openly about their feelings, people may avoid looking at the mastectomy, and the emotional wound may continue to exist long after the physical wound has healed. It is important for any woman to become comfortable with these body changes as soon as possible and to involve her partner. Many resources are available to help. Check the bibliography for books such as *Spinning Straw into Gold*, or *Man to Man, for the Husband of the Woman with Breast Cancer*. Support groups, other patients, your medical caregivers, and counselors are all resources to help you find ways to discuss this important issue with your partner.

Sexuality, self-esteem and femininity are important issues that affect women undergoing treatment for breast cancer. You may be experiencing hormonal changes and menopausal symptoms that result from the chemotherapy or hormonal therapy. It is very important for you to communicate your questions and feelings to your physician, nurse, or your partner. Discussing your feelings with your partner and expressing your desire for physical affection are necessary for maintaining closeness. Let your partner know that direct communication is important for you.

At this time you may be focused on your needs, your treatment and its side effects. Your partner may experience this as a withdrawal. Remember you are both coping with a shift in roles as you adjust to many changes. You may have feelings of insecurity and guilt. Experiencing these difficult feelings is a normal part of the coping process. Openly addressing and discussing feelings and fears with a counselor or support group can help in coping with emotional and physical changes associated with breast cancer treatment. Allow yourself time to adapt to the changes in your body, your self image and your feelings about yourself, and to reestablish physical intimacy with your partner.

Support Groups

Many cancer patients find strength and support through sharing their thoughts and feelings with other women who have been through a common experience. Support groups can be helpful for deriving emotional support and sharing information.

Support groups, frequently led by knowledgeable professionals, often include an educational focus as well as offering the opportunity for open discussions. It is important to remember that every person is different and that a treatment given to one person may not be appropriate for another. Also remember that responses to treatment will differ, so that the experience of others with similar disease is not necessarily predictive of what you will experience.

When looking for a support group, ask your nurse, social worker or doctor about available programs in your area. It is also recommended that you call first to confirm format, times and other information.

Breast Cancer Support Groups

Greater Seattle Area

Evergreen Cancer Center
12303 NE 130th Lane, Suite 120
Kirkland, WA 98034
Wellness Works — Bosom Buddies
Jacqui Dodge, (425) 899-2264

Highline Hospital
16251 Sylvester Rd. SW
Burien, WA 98166
Eileen Stein, (206) 244-9970, x5249

Northwest Hospital
1560 N. 115th St.
Seattle, WA 98133
Breast Cancer Support Group
Liz White, RN, (206) 368-1299

A Healing Place: Support and sharing while coping with advanced breast disease.
Suzane Kirsch, M.A.
(206) 642-4034

Overlake Hospital
1035 116th NE
Bellevue, WA 98004
Carol Mickley, (425) 747-4988
Suzie Hughes, (425) 481-0490

Providence Comprehensive Breast Center
1600 E. Jefferson, Suite 300
Seattle, WA 98122
Susan Leavitt, MSW, (206) 320-4341

Seattle Area Breast Cancer Support Group
St. Stephen's Episcopal Church
4805 NE 45th St.
Seattle, WA 98006
Tath Hossfeld, (425) 774-0313
Jonelle Dedrick, (206) 784-9697

Group Health
Group Health Central
200 16th Ave. East
Seattle, WA 98112
"Living With Cancer"
(206) 326-3440

Seattle Lesbian Cancer Project
1122 E. Pike St.
Seattle, WA 98122
(206) 323-6540

Team Survivor Northwest
200 N.E. Pacific, Suite 101
Seattle, WA 98195
Health education and fitness programs for all women affected by cancer.
Julia Cañas, (206) 732-8350

Swedish Tumor Institute
1225 Madison
Seattle, WA 98104
(206) 386-2323 *
*Ask operator for recorded message for support group dates and times.

UWMC Breast Care Cancer Research Center
1959 N.E. Pacific
Box 356043
Seattle, WA 98195
www.UWBreastcancer.com

Support and education group for women recently diagnosed with breast cancer; ongoing group and support group for patients with recurrent and/or metastatic breast cancer.
Meghan Anderson, (206) 598-4456
Susan Keller, (206) 598-4527

High Risk & Genetics Support Group
Ksenia Peters, MS, (206) 616-4293

Living Well with Cancer series:
educational events and classes for cancer patients and caregivers.
Janet Parker, (206) 598-7880

Puget Sound Tumor Institute
21601 76ᵗʰ Ave. W.
Edmonds, WA 98026
Melanie Reynolds
(425) 640-4306

"Circle of Friends" Women of Color Breast Support Group
Central and South Seattle Areas
Call Kim Taylor for locations
(206) 461-6900, ext. 203

Providence General Medical Center
Pacific Campus
916 Pacific Ave.
Everett, WA 98201
Patti Davis, CSW, (425) 258-7255

Valley Medical Center
400 S. 43ʳᵈ , Renton WA 98055
"I Can Cope" and "Look Good, Feel Better" classes offered during year; call for dates and times.
Connie Grace, (425) 656-4002

Virginia Mason Medical Center
925 Seneca
Seattle, WA 98111
"Living With Cancer" support group/educational series for patients, families, friends and the community.
Ann McElroy, (206) 583-6541
Josie Stevenson, (206) 583-6578

North Puget Sound

North Puget Sound Oncology Clinic
1415 E. Kincaid
Mt. Vernon, WA 98273
Support group and Living with Cancer series
Ruth Mora, (360) 416-8418

Bellingham Breast Center
2940 Squalicum Pkwy
Bellingham, WA 98225
"The Next Step" support group
(360) 671-9688

Island Hospital (Burrows Room)
Anacortes, WA 98221
Breast Cancer Support Group
Deborah Mc Intosh, (360) 293-4745

Whidbey General Hospital
Breast Cancer Support Group
Renee Yanke, ARNP
(360) 321-5173 (South Whidbey)
(360) 678-7624 (North Whidbey)

South Puget Sound Area

Madigan Army Medical Center
General Cancer Support Group
Patty Berke, MSW, (253) 968-0753

GANTS
American RedCross
Tacoma, WA 98431
Betty Carlson, (253) 968-1055

Encore Aquatic Exercises Peer Support Group, YWCA
405 Broadway
Tacoma, WA 98402
(253) 272-4181

Tacoma General Hospital
315 S. Martin Luther King Way
Tacoma, WA 98405

Breast Cancer Support Group
Oncology, (253) 403-1677

Cancer, a Course of Hope
Pat Carpenter, (253) 552-1011

United Methodist Church
1322 3rd Street S.E.
Puyallup, WA 98372
Sue Yamani, (253) 841-4297

Community Breast Cancer Awareness Center, Circle of Friends
Long Term Survivor Support Group
4002 S. 12th St.
Tacoma, WA 98405
(253) 752-4222

Kitsap/Pierce Peninsula

Gig Harbor Breast Cancer Support Group
United Methodist Church
Sund Fellowship Room
7400 Pioneer Way
Gig Harbor, WA 98335
Kay Musgrove, RNC, (253) 857-5802
kmusgrov@linknet.lib.wa.us

Harrison Hospital
2520 Cherry Ave.
Bremerton, WA 98310
Kay Buitenveld, (360) 792-6885

Clark County

Cancer Center of Southwest Washington Medical Center
400 N.E. Mother Joseph Pl.
Vancouver, WA 98644
Breast Cancer Education Support Group, (360) 514-2174

Southeastern Washington

Tri-Cities Cancer Center Breast Cancer Support Group
7350 West Deschutes Avenue
Kennewick, WA 99336
Julie Gregory, (509) 737-3374
Kathy Leonard, (509) 545-9816

Central Washington

Women's Cancer Support Group
Wellness House
210 S. 11ᵗʰ Ave., Suite 40
Yakima, WA 98902
(509) 575-6686

Pullman Memorial Hospital
Breast Cancer Support Group
Darlene Ames, (509) 336-0291

Support Groups for Family Members and Friends

Evergreen Hospital Medical Center
12040 N.E. 128th
Kirkland WA 98034
Childrens' Support Group (ages 6-12)
Teenagers' Support Group
Judy Jones, (425) 899-2264

Northwest Hospital
1550 N 115ᵗʰ St.
Seattle, WA 98133
"Living With Cancer — Friends and Family." Support group for friends and family members of cancer patients.
Roeliena VanZanten, (206) 368-1598

Bastyr Natural Health Clinic
Cancer Support Group
1307 N. 45ᵗʰ St.
For families and friends of patients with cancer.
Dr. Keith Grieneeks, (206) 834-4155

Other Support Services

Cancer Lifeline
6522 Fremont Avenue North
Seattle, WA 98103-5358
Offers free services for cancer patients and caregivers, including relaxation and visualization series, nutrition classes, 24-hour lifeline, family support program, kids' group, exercise workshop and yoga.
(206) 297-2100 or (800) 255-5505
24 hour lifeline: (206) 297-2500
www.cancerlifeline.org

Evergreen Cancer Center
12303 NE 130th Lane, Suite 120
Kirkland, WA 98034
Childrens' Support Group and Teenagers' Support Group
Jacqui Dodge, (425) 899-2264

Touched by Cancer
Judy Jones, (425) 899-2264

℘RESOURCES

Books

Lange, V., M.D. Be a Survivor: Your Guide to Breast Cancer Treatment (Lange Productions, 1998)

Stoppard, M. The Breast Book (DK Publishing, Inc., 1996)

Swirsky, J., and Balaban, B. The Breast Cancer Handbook: Taking Control After You Have Found a Lump (Power Publishers, 1998)

Wittman, J. Breast Cancer Journal: A Century of Petals (Fulcrum Pub., 1993)

McCarthy, P., and Loren, J.A., editors. Breast Cancer? Let Me Check My Schedule! (Westview Press, 1993)

Hirshaut, Y., M.D., and Pressman, P., M.D. Breast Cancer: The Complete Handbook (Bantam, 1996)

Altman, R., and Sarg, M., M.D. The Cancer Dictionary (Facts On File, 1992) (800) 322-8755

Lorde, A. The Cancer Journals (Aunt Lute Books, 1980)

Lauersen, N., M.D., Ph.D., and Stukane, E. The Complete Book of Breast Care (Fawcett Columbine, 1996)

Ploski, C. Conversations with My Healers - My Journey to Wellness from Breast Cancer (Council Oak Books, 1995)

Strauss, L. Coping When a Parent Has Cancer (Rosen Pub. Co., 1988)

Seirsky, J., R.N., and Sackett, D. Coping with Lymphedema (Avery Publishing Group, 1998)

Love, S., M.D., and Lindsey, K. Dr. Susan Love's Breast Book (Addison Wesley, 1995)

Wilber, K. Grace and Grit: Spirituality and Healing in the Life and Death of Treya Killam Wilber (Shambala Publications, 1993)

Mayer, L., editor. Holding Tight, Letting Go: Living with Metastatic Breast Cancer (O'Reilley and Assoc., 1997)

Porter, M. Hope is Contagious: The Breast Cancer Treatment Survival Handbook (Simon & Schuster, 1997)

Weiss, M., M.D. Living Beyond Breast Cancer: Survivor's Guide for When Treatment Ends And the Rest of Your Life Begins (Times Books, Random House, 1999)

Brack, P. and Brack, B. Moms Don't Get Sick (Melius Pub., 1990) (800) 882-5171

Clifford, C. Not Now...I'm Having a No Hair Day: Humor and Healing for People with Cancer (Pfeifer-Hamilton, 1996)

Conway, K. Ordinary Life: A Memoir of Illness (W.H.Freeman and Co., 1997)

Brinker, N. The Race Is Run One Step at a Time: My Personal Struggle and Every Woman's Guide to Taking Charge of Breast Cancer (Summit Publishing Group, 1995)

Kaye, R. Spinning Straw into Gold (Simon & Schuster, 1991)

Yalof, I. Straight From the Heart: Letters of Hope and Inspiration from Survivors of Breast Cancer (Kensington Books, 1996)

Fore, R. Survivors Guide to Breast Cancer: One Couple's Story of Faith, Hope and Love (Smyth & Helwys Publishing, Inc., 1998)

Virag, I.We're All in This Together: Families Facing Breast Cancer (Andrews and McMeel, 1995)

Lovert, S. When Someone You Love Has Cancer (Dell Pub. Co, 1995)

Feldman, G.You Don't Have To Be Your Mother (WW Norton & Co, 1994)

Borysenko, J. Minding the Body, Mending the Mind (Addison Wesley, 1987)

Cantor, R.C. And a Time to Live: Toward Emotional Well-being during the Crisis of Cancer (Harper and Row, 1978)

Capossela, C.,and Warnock, S. Share the Care (Fireside, 1995)

Cooke, M.,and Putman, E. Ways You Can Help (Warner Books, 1996)

Cousins, N. Anatomy of an Illness: As Perceived by the Patient (Bantam Books, 1981)

Cousins, N. The Healing Heart (Avon, 1983)

Dackman, L. Affirmations, Meditations, and Encouragements for Women Living with Breast Cancer (Diane Publishing, 1999) Available from the publisher, call (610) 499-7415

Daxter, C. Love and Peace through Affirmation (H.J. Kramer, 1989)

Donald, C. Someone I Love has Cancer (Catherine McCormick Donald Foundation, P.O. Box 51, Fredonia, WI 53021. FAX (414) 692-9585. 1-10 copies $2.50 each for shipping)

Fine, J. Afraid to Ask: A Book for Families to Share about Cancer (Lothrop, Lee and Shepard Books, 1986)

Fiore, N.A. The Road Back to Health: Coping with the Emotional Side of Cancer (Bantam Books, 1986)

Gawain, S. Creative Visualization (Bantam Books, 1978)

Harwell, A. When Your Friend Gets Cancer (Harold Shaw Publishers, 1987)

Hay, L. You Can Heal your Life (Hay House, 1988)

Johnson, J. Intimacy: Living as a Woman after Cancer (NC Press, 1987)

Jaffee, D.T. Healing from Within: Psychological Techniques to Help the Mind Heal the Body (Simon and Schuster, 1986)

Kievman, B., and Blackmun, S. For Better or Worse: A Couple's Guide to Dealing with Chronic Illness (Contemporary Books, 1989)

Le Shan, E. When a Parent is Very Sick (Atlantic Monthly Press, 1986)

Mullen, F. ,and Hoffman B. Charting the Journey (Consumer Reports, 1990)

Photopulos, G. Of Tears and Triumphs (Congdon & Weed, 1988)

Pomeroy, D. When Someone You Love Has Cancer (IBS Press, 1991)

Rossman, M.L. Healing Yourself: A Step-By-Step Program for Better Health Through Imagery (Pocket Books, 1984)

Siegel, B. Love, Medicine, & Miracles: Lessons Learned about Self-healing from a Surgeon's Experience with Exceptional Patients (Harper and Row, 1986)

Simonton, O.C., Matthews-Simonton, S., and Creighton, J. Getting Well Again: A Step-by-step Self-help Guide to Overcoming Cancer for Patients and Their Families (St. Martin's Press, 1978)

Strauss, L.L. Coping When a Parent Has Cancer (Rosen Publishing Co., 1988)

Publications

American Cancer Society. Helping Children Understand: A Guide for A Parent With Cancer (800) 227-2345

American Cancer Society. It Helps To Have Friends When Mom Or Dad Has Cancer (800) 227-2345

American Cancer Society. Breast Cancer Facts and Figures (1997, (800) 227-2345)

National Cancer Institute. When Someone in Your Family has Cancer (NCI Pub. No. 92-2685, (800) 422-6237)

National Cancer Institute. Taking Time: Support for People with Cancer and the People Who Care About Them (NCI Pub. No. 92-2059, (800) 422-6237)

Strauss, L. What About Me? A Booklet for Teenage Children of Cancer Patients (Cancer Family Care, 1986, (513) 731-3346)

Y-ME. When the Woman You Love Has Breast Cancer (1995, (312) 986-0020)

American Cancer Society. Sexuality and Cancer: For the Woman Who Has Cancer and Her Partner (800) 227-2345

Susan G. Komen Cancer Foundation. What's Happening to Me? Coping and Living With Breast Cancer (800) 462-9273

Susan G. Komen Cancer Foundation. What's Happening to Mom? Helping Children Cope With BreastCancer (800) 462-9273

Susan G. Komen Cancer Foundation. What's Happening to the Women We Love? Families Coping With Breast Cancer (800) 462-9273

Videos

American Cancer Society. A Significant Journey: Breast Cancer Survivors and the Men Who Love Them (800) 227-2345

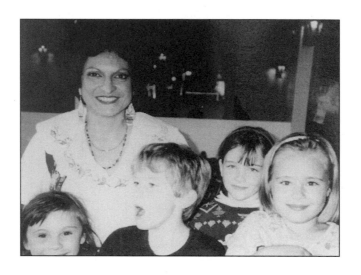

Patty Loveless
Diagnosed: Age 48, 1995

Peru, South America, is my birthplace. I am married and have one daughter and one son. In the middle of my chemotherapy, I wrote a poem I would like to share. It is about my feelings of war with cancer, and the strength I felt coming from God. It also reflects upon the good memories I have of my father and mother, who passed away before me.

> *Full enjoyment every second of your life,*
> *Put the bad things on your back,*
> *And kick them out with a laugh.*

17

Menopause Without Hormones

Chemotherapy often causes the sudden onset of menopause. Although estrogen replacement therapy is used in the general menopausal population, estrogen support for breast cancer survivors is controversial and not recommended by most oncologists. Women may struggle as they try to find ways to manage the associated side effects. Hot flashes, sleep disturbances, mood swings and vaginal dryness are obvious symptoms that women report, while osteoporosis and heart disease are silent, yet important, stalkers.

The following suggestions may help ease the side effects of menopause. As always, it is recommended that you review these suggested activities with your health care providers to ensure they are right for you.

Dealing with Hot Flashes and Night Sweats

Hot flashes are sudden, intense episodes in which the skin surface heats up and sweating occurs to cool the body down. They can happen during the day or at night, and vary in frequency and severity from woman to woman.

Life style changes to manage hot flashes include:

Avoid symptom triggers: Strong emotions, caffeine, alcohol, cayenne or other spices, tight clothing and hot weather can trigger reactions.

Exercise: Walk, swim, dance, bicycle, or row — 20 to 30 minutes each day.

Stay cool: Use well-ventilated rooms and fans. Dress in layers made of natural fabrics. Drink at least eight glasses of cool water per day.

Reduce your stress: Try deep, slow abdominal breathing, 6-8 breaths per minute. Practice for 15 minutes morning and evening, and use the technique whenever you feel a flash coming on.

Consider daily meditation, prayer, Tai Chi or yoga.

Eat food high in soy: Tofu, tempeh, and textured vegetable protein (TVP) are all good sources of soy. There are questions regarding high phytoestrogen intake for women whose tumors are hormone-receptor positive. Potential stimulation of tumor growth may occur, although this has not been well-studied scientifically. Modest amounts, e.g. occasional soy products, may be safer for this group of breast cancer patients.

Although more research is needed in the area of alternative approaches, the following list contains treatment for menopausal symptoms. Check with your provider before using. Some of these herbs contain phytoestrogens.

- Chinese herbs

- Accupuncture

- Vitamin E

- Bioflavinoids (plant estrogens)

- Garden sage (Salvia officinalis)

- Motherswort (Leonurrus cardiaca)

Western treatments include:

- Medroxy progesterone (Megace). A hormone sometimes used in high doses to treat breast cancer. At lower doses it can help hot flashes. Weight gain can be side effect.

- Bellergal. A combination of drugs which includes belladonna. Can help alleviate hot flashes, but sedation can be a bothersome side effect.

- Clonidine. A blood pressure medication which comes as a pill or a patch. Low blood pressure can be a side effect.

Menopausal Insomnia

Continual interruption of sleep makes life difficult. Night sweats and a racing heart associated with menopause can wake you up at night, and other factors can keep you from going back to sleep easily. Following the previous suggestions for dealing with hot flashes can help. In addition:

- Use bed linens made of natural fabric.

- Keep the bedroom temperature at 64-66 degrees.

- Avoid caffeine, excess alcohol and simple sugars (candy, cake) before bedtime. Caffeine and alcohol use can affect some individuals' sleep for days after consumption.

- Think of your bedroom as your place for peace, relaxation and sleep.

- Try to leave work and other discussions in the office or other rooms of your home.

- Stress counseling can be a helpful strategy when dealing with insomnia.

- Take a warm shower or bath at bedtime or after waking during your sleep time .

- Try to develop a routine of going to bed and getting up at the same times of day. If you have not fallen asleep after 20-30 minutes, get up and leave the bedroom.

Complementary treatments for insomnia can include:

- Chamomile tea

- Oatstraw

- Nettle tea

- Valerian (Valeriana officinalis), although it can be habit forming.

Western treatments for insomnia generally include drugs in the class called benzodiazepines. These medications are very good at inducing sleep, but have side effects that include prolonged drowsiness and the development of drug tolerance or addiction. Drugs in this class include: diazepam (Valium), alprazolam (Xanax), triazolam (Halcion), temazepam (Restoril), and zolpidem (Ambien).

Dealing with Mood Swings, Fears and Despair

• Stay connected to your community and nourish your friendships.

• Get involved with a support group or a counselor.

• Avoid tranquilizers.

• Find and practice activities that renew your spirit and your tranquility (relaxation exercises, prayer, meditation, yoga, and/or slow abdominal breathing).

• Consider using homeopathic remedies. Use a naturopath to guide you in their use.

Sexuality

When ovarian production of estrogen stops or is significantly decreased, all areas of the body stimulated by estrogen undergo some change. Women may notice a decreased sex drive and an increase in vaginal dryness, which can lead to pain with penetration of the vagina.

The ability to feel pleasure from touching almost always remains. Nerves and muscles involved in the sensation of orgasm (climax) are not lost because of menopause. There are very few medications that interfere with the nerves and muscles involved in orgasm.

Keep an open mind about ways to feel sexual pleasure. Menopause may give you and your partner an opportunity to learn new ways to give and receive satisfaction. Strive to maintain open communication with your partner about the changes that are taking place. In addition:

• Take time to relax and become aroused.

• Be sensitive to your level of energy. If you are too tired at the end of the day, consider making time with your partner at an earlier time in the day.

• Create an environment that enhances your sensuality and sexuality. Consider the effects of lighting, clothing, aromas, warmth and coolness.

If sexual problems persist, be sure to talk to your health care provider. Talk openly with him/her, and have a thorough pelvic exam. Counseling and support groups can help you and your partner develop better communication and reestablish your enjoyment of sexual intimacy.

Vaginal Dryness

The drop in estrogen levels at menopause can cause a decrease in the lubrication of the vagina. At the same time, the vaginal lining thins and becomes more fragile.

• Avoid chemical or mechanical irritants like feminine hygiene products.

• Keep sexually active.

• Apply a small amount of Vitamin E oil to the vagina to prevent the wicking away of your natural moisture.

• Try water-soluble lubricants for vaginal penetration. *Astroglide, Slippery Stuff, Imagination, Gyne-moisten*, and *K-Y* type gels are examples of these products. *Replens* adheres to the vaginal wall and is intended to last longer.

Vaginal estrogen is sometimes prescribed, but breast cancer survivors should ask about the amount of estrogen absorbed into the blood stream. Only a very small amount (a dab) is needed for the relief of vaginal dryness. A low-dose estrogen ring, *Estring*, is less messy than creams and is minimally absorbed into the rest of the body. Do not use estrogen creams as a lubricant.

Preventing Osteoporosis

Prevention and treatment of osteoporosis in breast cancer patients involve diet, exercise, and in some women, anti-osteoporotic medications. Osteoporosis is a thinning of the bones due to loss of bone minerals (mainly calcium). Estrogen protects women from bone loss, which accelerates after menopause. Estrogen is an excellent drug for the prevention and treatment of osteoporosis, although it is usually avoided in breast cancer patients.

The current calcium recommendation for women under 65 is 1000 mg per day when estrogen or other osteoporosis preventive medications are used. Otherwise, 1,500 mg per day is recommended.

Calcium-dense foods include dairy products, calcium-fortified orange juice and fortified soymilk. Very dark green vegetables and dried beans contain calcium in smaller amounts. A large variety of calcium supplements are on the market.

Vitamin D is necessary for the body to absorb and use calcium. Current recommendations are 400 IU per day until age 70, then 800 IU. In addition, magnesium at about half the dosage of calcium helps your body utilize the calcium.

The bisphosphonate called alendronate (Fosamax) and the anti-estrogen raloxifene (Evista) have been approved by the FDA to treat and/or prevent osteoporosis. It is well recognized that tamoxifen (Nolvadex), commonly used in the treatment of breast cancer, also has a protective effect against bone mineral loss. Several other drugs are currently under investigation.

Exercise is also important in building and maintaining premenopausal bone mass and improving balance. Choose types that are muscle building and put reasonable stress on your bones. You may want to consider working with a physical therapist, exercise physiologist or other provider to develop a safe, effective plan.

Preventing Heart Disease

Post-menopausal women who are not on hormone replacement therapy are generally at a higher risk of heart disease. Take care of yourself by developing and maintaining a routine with at least 20-30 minutes per day of moderate exercise; it can be 10-15 minutes at a time. Walk, climb stairs, bicycle, dance, swim or row. Joining an organized aerobics program can sometimes provide the motivation and support to keep you in a program.

- Stop smoking. Smoking triples the risk of heart disease.

- Eat a wide variety of vegetables, fruits and whole grains, including soy foods, every day.

- Prepare food without frying or adding excessive amounts of oil.

- Read the labels on your food products. Avoid items with high fat and cholesterol content.

- Try to limit your diet to 20 grams or less of saturated fat per day.

- The B vitamins also have a role in decreasing heart disease.

- Being 20 percent or more overweight increases your risk of heart disease.

✍RESOURCES

Books

Barbach, L. The Pause: Positive Approaches to Menopause (Penguin Books, 1993)

Greenwood, S. Menopause Naturally: Preparing for the Second Half of Your Life (Volcano Press, 3rd edition, 1992)

Lark, S. The Menopause Self-Help Book (Celestial Arts, 1998)

Love, S., and Lindsey, K. Dr. Susan Love's Hormone Book: Making Informed Choices About Menopause (Times Books, 1998)

Roth, D. "No, It's Not Hot in Here": A Husband's Guide to Understanding Menopause (Ant Hill Press, 1999)

Saten, R., Borwaht, M., and Gleason, S. Menopause: Treatment Options for Women Surviving Breast Cancer or Concerned about Estrogen Replacement (The Hormone Foundation, 1997)

Sheehy, G. The Silent Passage (Random House, 1991)

Taylor, D., and Sumrall, A. Women of the 14th Moon: Writings on Menopause (Crossing Press, 1991)

Weed, S. Breast Cancer? Breast Health: The Wise Woman's Ways (Ash Tree, 1996)

Newsletters

A Friend Indeed: For Women in the Prime of Life (Box 1710, Champlain, NY 12919-1710)

Hot Flash: Newsletter for Midlife and Older Women (Box 816, Stony Brook, NY 11790-0609)

Menopause Management (Pamela J. Boggs, publisher, P.O. Box 658, Flanders, NJ 07856) This bimonthly, endorsed by the North American Menopause Society, provides practical clinical guidelines — not research findings — on management of women's health during and after menopause.

Menopause News (2074 Union St., San Francisco, CA 94123)

Harvard Women's Health Watch (Harvard Medical School Health Publications Group, 164 Longwood Ave, Boston, MA 02115)

Nutrition Action Health Letter (Center for Science in the Public Interest, Suite 300, 1875 Connecticut Ave. NW, Washington, DC 20009-5728)

University of California, Berkeley, Wellness Letter (PO Box 359162, Palm Court, FL 32035)

Organizations

The North American Menopause Society
P.O. Box 94527
Cleveland, Ohio 44101
(440) 442-7550, (800) 774-5342

National Women's Health Network (NWHN)
514 10th Street N.W., Suite 400
Washington, DC 20004
(202) 347-1140

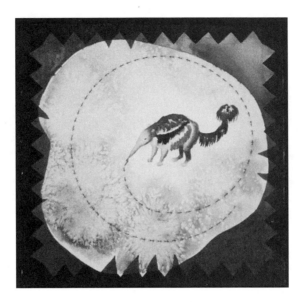

Sharon Hines-Pinion

Healing Visualization: My Friend Herbie Eats Cancer Cells ⇘ Watercolor

18

The Financial, Insurance and Legal Impact of Breast Cancer

Financial Options

Resources are available for uninsured and underinsured women who have health insurance and other financial difficulties. Residents of Washington state are eligible for public assistance depending on their financial resources. To obtain more information or to apply for assistance, contact a local Community Service Office (CSO). If you have difficulty locating that office, contact the Medical Assistance Administration at (800) 562-3022 to ask for help.

The Basic Health Plan, a low-cost package of benefits, is available to individuals and businesses across the state. The plan is available at full cost to anyone, although the system often has a waiting list for enrollment. A sliding scale is used to adjust premiums for low-income individuals and families. For information about the Basic Health Plan, including specific benefits and costs, contact the Basic Health Plan at (800) 826-2444.

To get answers to questions regarding Medicare eligibility and enrollment, contact the Social Security Administration at (800) 772-1213.

All hospitals have some money provided by the federal government under the Hill-Burton Act to provide care to individuals with no health insurance. Women can contact the patient financial office, patient referral line, or patient advocate provided by their hospital to find out about alternative resources for health care coverage.

Pharmaceutical companies have needs-based programs. The American Cancer Society and Y-Me are examples of nonprofit community groups that provide free services in such areas as transportation, prostheses, wigs and skin care.

℗FINANCIAL RESOURCES

Organizations

American Cancer Society
(800) 227-2345
Services: Provides prostheses, wigs, transportation and limited other
financial assistance on a case by case basis.

Basic Health Plan
Washington State Health Care Authority
(800) 826-2444
676 Woodland Square Loop S.E.
P.O. Box 42682
Olympia, WA 98504-2682

Community Service Offices

Washington State Department of Social and Health Services
(425) 775-5555
Look in the governmental pages of your local telephone book under "State
Government; Social and Health Services; Community Services Office" for
closest location.
Services: Provides Medicaid, food stamps and short-term disability
financial assistance.

Directory of Prescription Drug Patient Assistance Programs
800-PMA-INFO [(800) 762-4636]
www.phrma.org
Services: Provides listings of drug companies that provide prescription
medicines free of charge to physicians whose patients might not
otherwise have access to necessary medicines.

National Coalition for Cancer Survivorship (NCCS)
1010 Wayne Avenue, Suite 505
Silver Spring, MD 20910-5600
(888) 650-9127; www.cansearch.org
Services: Serves as a clearinghouse for information and materials on
survivorship and acts as an advocate for cancer survivors, especially in
employment, insurance and health care reform.

Social Security Administration
(800) 772-1213
Services: A toll-free hotline with representatives available to answer questions regarding Medicare benefits.

Washington State Department of Social and Health Services
Medical Assistance Administration
617 8th Ave SE
Olympia, WA 98504
(800) 562-3022
Services: To maximize opportunities for low-income people to obtain appropriate, quality health services.

Insurance Coverage

Federal and State laws govern private health insurance. The rules of your health insurance plan are dependent on whether you purchase it yourself (individual plan) or it is purchased by your employer (group health plan), or you are part of a self-funded plan. A self-funded health plan is exempt from State regulations. State regulations will entitle you to certain kinds of coverage.

Breast cancer-related State of Washington mandatory health benefits are:

• **Mammography Screening.** Disability policies covering hospital and medical expenses must cover mammography screening or diagnostic services.

• **Mastectomy.** No insurer may cancel or deny coverage or restrict the rates or benefits of a person who received a mastectomy or lumpectomy more than 5 years previously.

• **Breast Reconstruction.** Disability policies covering hospital and medical expenses must cover breast reconstruction resulting from mastectomy.

In 1996, Congress passed the Health Insurance Portability and Accountability Act (HIPAA). This law and Washington's health insurance laws protect you in purchasing health insurance, or if you have a serious health condition.

In Washington, your health insurance options do not depend on your health status. All health plans in Washington must limit the exclusion of preexisting conditions. Your health insurance can not be cancelled because you are sick. An individual health plan can not turn you down for coverage because of your age or health status.

Health insurance can be categorized in two types of coverage: indemnity plans and managed care. Within the two types of coverage there are four types of plans: fee for service, Preferred Provider Organizations (PPO), Point of Service plans (POS) and Health Maintenance Organizations (HMO). No one type of health insurance is better than the other. The differences among the types of health insurance are related to your costs and how you access care. It is important to understand what type of health care coverage you have and the access rules and costs associated with it.

The place to start in understanding your health insurance coverage is your benefit booklet or Certificate of Coverage. The customer service department of your health insurance company will also be able to answer questions related to your benefits.

SHIBA (Statewide Health Insurance Benefits Advisors) is a statewide network of trained volunteers who help consumers and their families with questions about health insurance. The Washington State Insurance Commissioner's Office sponsors this free service. Volunteers in communities around the state are available to meet with consumers to discuss Medicare, Medigap (Medicare Supplement) insurance, managed care, long-term care insurance, employment-related benefits, medical billings assistance, and other consumer protection issues. You can reach the toll-free SHIBA referral line at (800) 397-4422 to set up an interview with a SHIBA volunteer.

In filing a claim or disputing a denied claim, there are some general tips which may help:

- Review your policy or employee benefit booklet carefully to be sure the service in question is covered.

- Follow any managed care rules, including precertification requirements and use of network providers.

- If a claim is denied, the reason for the denial should be stated on your Explanation of Benefits.

- If you disagree with the denial, check your policy or employee benefit booklet for the insurance company's appeal process.

- The company should be able to answer questions regarding the appeal process over the telephone.

• Your appeal should be in writing, and it may be necessary to provide information from your doctor. Be sure to keep copies of your appeal.

If you have tried unsuccessfully to resolve a claim dispute with your insurance company, you may need to contact the Washington State Insurance Commissioner's office. The Insurance Complaints Division can be reached at (800) 562-6900. The staff will be able to advise you how to file a complaint with their office.

Currently people 65 or older, and people with qualifying disabilities, are eligible for Medicare. Certain women with advanced breast cancer may qualify under Medicare's disability eligibility. To get answers to questions regarding Medicare eligibility and enrollment, contact the Social Security Administration at (800) 772-1213. It is important to ask whether your provider accepts Medicare claims before service.

Medicaid is a joint state and federal health insurance program for low-income individuals with medical needs. Applications for Medicaid are made through your local Community Service Office of the Washington State Department of Social and Health Services. It is advisable to make sure your provider accepts Medicaid reimbursement payments before being seen.

In 1993 the Family and Medical Leave Act (FLMA) was signed into law. It guarantees that people who work for companies with more than 50 employees can take up to 12 weeks' unpaid leave a year to care for a newborn or newly adopted child, or for certain seriously ill family members, or to recover from their own serious health conditions. To find out more about this law, contact your employer's Human Resources Department or the Labor Department's Wage and Hour Division at 111 Third Ave., Suite 755, Seattle, WA 98101-3212, (206) 553-4482.

℘ INSURANCE RESOURCES

Selected articles, books and pamphlets

Buying Health Insurance (Washington State Insurance Commission, updated regularly) (800) 753-7300, (800) 562-6900

"Dealing with Insurance Problems" (In The Breast Cancer Handbook, by Swirsky, J., and Barbara, B., Power Publications,1998)

"Insurance" (In The Breast Cancer Companion by La Tour, K., Avon Books,1994)

"Managing Insurance Issues" (In Facing Forward, A Guide for Cancer Survivors (National Coalition for Cancer Survivorship, 1999) (888) 650-9127

Organizations

Health Insurance Association of America
555 13th Street NW
Washington, DC 20004
(202) 824-1600
www.hiaa.org
Services: Publishes several manuals on health and disability insurance.

Washington State Insurance Commission
Consumer Advocacy and Outreach Division
(800) 562-6900
P.O. Box 40256
Olympia, WA 98504-0256
Services: Advises and advocates for consumers experiencing problems with group and individual insurance policies related to contract compliance and state laws. Provides information over the telephone. Does not have jurisdiction over self-insured plans, which are not regulated under federal laws.

Legal

Legal issues related to breast cancer typically fall into two general areas: 1) those involving employment, insurance and public benefits, and 2) those involving basic legal matters affecting your assets and health care wishes.

Employment, insurance and public benefits

If disputes arise regarding employment, insurance, and public benefits, they typically require independent analysis of the facts and review of applicable violations of laws. The type of legal assistance needed depends on the issues being raised and the type of remedies sought. When seeking legal advice, be prepared to provide a clear description of the problem with appropriate documentation to support your position.

Finding appropriate legal counsel can be challenging. It is rare to find an attorney, or legal group, with special experience related to breast cancer. Fortunately, many attorneys have had experience with employment discrimination and insurance coverage issues. The Northwest Women's Law Center and county bar associations provide referrals. People with limited income may contact the Northwest Justice Project for assistance.

It is always advisable to seek legal assistance prior to filing a complaint, since many legal complaints must follow state and/or federal filing guidelines. These guidelines may require adherence to strict timelines. In some cases, complaints must be filed with government agencies prior to taking other legal actions. For example, employment discrimination complaints must first be filed with the U.S. Department of Health and Human Service's Office of Civil Rights. When selecting an attorney, always ask about his/her experience with similar cases and the outcomes, and estimated costs.

Personal assets and health care wishes

Legal instruments are available to deal with matters involving personal assets and health care wishes. A basic list of legal instruments regarding health care wishes, legal and financial affairs and distribution of assets in the event of death would include:

- A Durable Power of Attorney for Health Care allows your designee to carry out your health care decisions if you become unable to do so yourself.

- A Durable Power of Attorney for Legal and Financial Affairs allows your designee to manage your legal and financial affairs if you are unable to do so yourself.

- A Health Care Directive outlines the medical procedures you may, or may not, want performed. These include tube feeding and life support machines.

- Wills are used to direct where and how your assets will be distributed when you die.

Forms are available at business stationery stores, some medical facilities, and private attorneys' offices, and many excellent books have been written to provide detailed information about each of these options.

⊗ LEGAL RESOURCES

Selected articles, books and pamphlets

American Cancer Society. Cancer and Employment Discrimination: Washington (ACS, 1989) (800) 227-2345, (800) 729-1151

Earning a Living – Facing Forward, a Guide for Cancer Survivors (National Coalition for Cancer Surviorship, 1999) (888) 650-9127

Organizations

Northwest Justice
401 2nd Ave. S., Suite 406
Seattle, WA, 98104
(206) 464-1519
Services: Provides free legal assistance to low-income people regarding public entitlements (e.g., Medicaid and food stamps).

Northwest Women's Law Center
119 So. Main St., Suite 410
Seattle, WA 98104-2515
(206) 621-7691 (Information and Referrals)
(206) 682-9552 (Administration)

Services: Provides legal information and referrals to private attorneys. Represents clients involved in impact litigation (i.e., litigation which may affect large groups of women, such as insurance coverage of bone marrow transplants for breast cancer).

Washington State Human Rights Commission
1511 3rd Ave., Suite 921
Melbourne Tower TB41
Seattle, WA 98101-1621
(206) 464-6500
Services: Provides information on filing discrimination complaints.

U.S. Department of Health and Human Services
Office for Civil Rights
2201 6th Ave.
Seattle, WA 98121
(206) 615-2288
Services: Provides information on filing discrimination complaints against companies receiving federal funds.

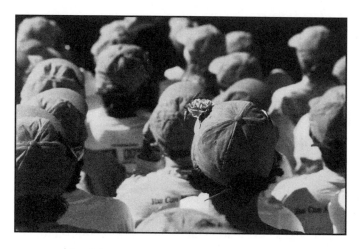

Patricia Krause ❧ *My Sisters* ❧ Photograph

19

Resources for Breast Cancer Patients

ℰℴ

Discovering that you have breast cancer can be a very lonely experience until you discover the many resources, organizations, and information sources that have been created to assist you. From national hotlines to local transportation assistance to personal accounts of the breast cancer journey, here is a listing of general resources you may find helpful. More specialized resources are listed later in this guide.

✆ RESOURCES

Local Hotlines

Cancer Lifeline
24-hour emotional support and resource referral for Washington state
(800) 255-5505
In King County: (206) 297-2500

CancerLink
Confidential telephone support for patients, families and caregivers from trained volunteers who have had a similar experience.
Voice mail: (425) 688-5266

National Hotlines

Cancer Hope Network

National one-to-one emotional support for patients and families undergoing chemotherapy and/or radiation treatment, from trained volunteers who have survived the treatments themselves.
877-HOPE-NET (467-3638)

Susan G. Komen Breast Cancer Foundation

For information on breast health or breast cancer concerns, call the National Toll-Free Breast Care Helpline at 800-I'M AWARE [(800) 462-9273]

National Cancer Institute's Cancer Information Service

Information in English or Spanish on treatment, clinical trials, advanced cancer, local services and dietary suggestions. Provides a computer printout called PDQ (Physicians' Data Query), updated monthly, on breast cancer and treatment options. 800-4-CANCER [(800) 422-6237]; cancernet.nei.nih.gov.

Share

Self-help for women with breast or ovarian cancer
1501 Broadway, Suite 1720, New York, NY 10036
Office: (212) 719-0364; Ovarian Cancer information: (212) 719-1204;
English hotline: (212) 382-2111; Spanish hotline: (212) 719-4454;
Fax: (212) 869-3431

National Breast Cancer Organization

24-hour hotline offering counseling for breast cancer patients, families and friends. (800) 221-2141

Y-ME: For Men with Breast Cancer

A male counselor most closely matched in experience to the caller will return a call within 24 hours.
(800) 221-2141; (312) 986-8228, Monday through Friday 7 a.m. to 3 p.m.

Breast Cancer Organizations

National Alliance of Breast Cancer Organizations (NABCO)
A nonprofit, national resource for information and advocacy for breast cancer patients. 9 East 37th Street, 10th Floor, New York, NY 10016. Information Services: www.nabco.org

National Breast Cancer Coalition
Active in obtaining increased funding for breast cancer research. 1707 "L" St. NW, Suite 1060, Washington, DC 20036. (202) 296-7477, www.natlbcc.org

Susan G. Komen Breast Cancer Foundation
An international organization with a mission to eradicate breast cancer as a life-threatening disease by advancing research, education, screening and treatment. For information on breast health or breast cancer concerns, call the Susan G. Komen Foundation's National toll-free Breast Care Helpline at (800) I'M AWARE (462-9273) or visit the Foundation's Website at www.breastcancerinfo.com. *Headquarters:* The Susan G. Komen Breast Cancer Foundation, 5005 LBJ Freeway, Suite 250, LB74, Dallas, TX 75244. (972) 855-1600. *Local Affiliate:* The Susan G. Komen Foundation, Puget Sound Affiliate, P.O. Box 85900, Seattle, WA 98145. (206) 633-0303; ww.seattlekomen.org, www.seattleraceforthecure.org, SGK.pskomen.org

Y-ME
National organization for breast cancer information, support and counseling for breast cancer patients and families. 212 W. Van Buren St., Chicago, IL 60607. (312) 986-8338 or 24-hour hotline (800) 221-2141 (English), (800) 986-9505 (Spanish). www.y-me.org

Wellness Works
Evergreen Hospital Medical Center
12040 N.E. 128th St.
Kirkland, WA 98034
(425) 899-2264
Information and support for people with

Cancer Organizations

American Cancer Society
Publications, information and emotional support . Information on
pharmaceutical company drug financial assistance programs. ACS programs
differ geographically, but may include I Can Cope (education), Reach to
Recovery (rehabilitation), Road to Recovery (transportation assistance), and
"Look Good...Feel Better" (grooming and appearance during treatment).
Patient services programs may include transportation reimbursement
housing. National information line: 800-ACS-2345; www.cancer.org.

> Western Pacific Division office: 2120 1st N., Seattle, WA 98109.
> (800) 729-1151, (206) 283-1152; www.cancer.org

> Southwest area: 1551 Broadway, Suite 200, Tacoma, WA 98402.
> (800) 729-3880, (253) 272-5767; www.cancer.org

Biological Therapy Institute Foundation
Resource for physician and patient information on biopharmaceuticals in
cancer therapy. P.O. Box 680429, Franklin, TN 37068. (615) 790-7535; Fax:
(615) 794-9110

Cancer Lifeline
Local organization providing emotional support and information about cancer-
related issues. Programs include family support program, workplace
consultation, kids'/parents group, movement awareness workshops, relaxation
and stress reduction series, pain management, and nutrition classes. Dorothy S.
O'Brien Center, 6522 Fremont Ave. N., Seattle, 98103. Program information:
(206) 297-2100. Hotline: (206) 297-2500 or (800) 255-5505 (toll-free in
Washington state); www.cancerlifeline.org

Chemotherapy Foundation
Supports laboratory and clinical research to develop more effective methods of
diagnosis and therapy for the control and cure of cancer. Conducts professional
and public education programs and provides free patient and public
information booklets. 183 Madison Avenue, Suite 403, New York, NY 10016.
(212) 213-9292; fax: (212) 213-3831.

Corporate Angel Network (CAN)
Helps cancer patients in stable condition travel between home and needed
treatment, using corporate aircraft. One Loop Road, Westchester County
Airport, White Plains, NY 10604, (914) 328-1313; Fax: (914) 328-3938; E-mail:
info@corpangelnetwork.org; Internet: www.corangelnetwork.org

National Cancer Survivors' Day (NCSD) Foundation
Sponsors celebration of life for cancer survivors, families, friends, and oncology teams on the first Sunday in June in communities throughout America. P.O. Box 682285, Franklin, TN 37068-2285. (615) 794-3006; Fax: (615) 794-0179; www.ncsdp.org

The National Coalition for Cancer Survivorship (NCCS)
Network of groups and individuals concerned with survivorship and resources for cancer patients and their families. A clearinghouse of information and advocacy for cancer survivors. 1010 Wayne Ave., 5th Floor, Silver Spring, MD 20910. (877) 622-7937 (toll-free); www.cansearch.org

Other Organizations and Resources

AirLifeline
National network of volunteer pilots who provide free air transportation for ambulatory patients. 50 Fullerton Court, Suite 200, Sacramento, CA 95825. (916) 641-7800 or toll-free (800) 446-1231; Fax: (916) 641-0600 (Monday through Friday, 7:30 a.m. to 4:30 p.m., Pacific Time); E-mail: staff@airlifeline.org; Internet: www.airlifeline.org

BreastDoctor.com
An internet site designed as an educational tool for breast cancer patients and their families. It is written, edited, and maintained by a group of physicians who specialize in breast cancer. Physicians who specialize in breast cancer care or have received special training in the surgical treatment of breast cancer are listed so that patients can find specialists close to their hometowns. Internet: www:breastdoctor.com/breast/doctor.htm

The Humor Project
A resource for humorous materials; free catalog. Holds conferences on use of humor in coping with illness. 480 Broadway, Suite 210, Saratoga Springs, NY 12866-2288. (518) 587-8770

Make Today Count
Mutual support for persons with life-threatening illnesses. c/o Connie Zimmerman, Mid-America Cancer Center, 1235 E. Cherokee, Springfield, MO 65804-2263. (800) 432-2273; Fax: (417) 888-7426

My Image After Breast Cancer Information and Support Group, Inc.
6000 Stevenson Ave., Suite 203, Alexandria, VA 22304
Hotline: (703) 461-9616 (Monday through Friday, 9 a.m. to 3 p.m. Eastern
time)

National Association of Hospital Hospitality Houses, Inc.
Information on lodging and support for families receiving medical care away
from home. 4013 W. Jackson St., Muncie, IN 47304 (800) 542-9730.
Fax: (317) 287-0321

National Family Caregivers Association
Membership organization dedicated to improving life for family caregivers
through information, publications, and education and public awareness
activities. Publishes a resource guide and a newsletter, and matches caregivers
for peer support. (800) 896-3650. E-mail: info@nfcares.org

National Patient Air Transport Hotline (NPATH)
Makes referrals to charitable organizations and special discounted patient
medical air transport services based on an evaluation of patient needs. P.O. Box
1940, Manassas, VA 22110. (800) 296-1217. Fax: (757) 412-4394.
E-mail: npathmsg@aol.com. Internet: www.npath.org

National Self-Help Clearinghouse
Makes referrals to regional self-help services, particularly regarding insurance
concerns and employment rights. 25 West 43rd St., Rm. 620, New York, NY
10036. (212) 817-1810

National Women's Health Network
Newsletters and position papers on women's health topics. 514 10th St. NW,
Suite 400, Washington, DC 20004. (202) 347-1140

Oncolink
University of Pennsylvania Cancer Center's online resource which provides
comprehensive information about specific types of cancer, updates on cancer
treatments and news about research advances. www.oncolink.upenn.edu/
disease/breast/

OnHealth.com
An independent online service that provides health and medical information
and resources. Includes a Breast Cancer Center, a breast cancer patient's diary,
and a breast cancer discussion group. www.onhealth.com/ch1/index.asp

Reach to Recovery
One-to-one visits by a breast cancer survivor to provide emotional support, information and exercise instruction. Sponsored by the American Cancer Society. 800-ACS-2345

The Wellness Community
Support and education programs encouraging emotional recovery and a feeling of wellness. All services are free. 2716 Ocean Park Boulevard, Suite 1040, Santa Monica, CA 90405. (310) 314-2555; Fax: (714) 660-9262

Other Local Resources

Community Breast Cancer Awareness Center (CBCAC)
Provides breast cancer information and resources, a "buddy" system for guidance and emotional support. Special programs and classes. 4002 South 12th St., Tacoma, WA 98405. (253) 752-4222; Fax: (253) 752-1202

Community Resources On-line (CRO)
Community Information Line (Monday through Friday, 8 a.m. to 6 p.m.): (206) 461-3200, or toll-free (800) 621-4636. 24-hour Crisis Line: (206) 461-3222 or toll-free (800) 244-5767. E-mail: info@crisisclinic.org. www.ci.seattle.wa.us/crisisclinic/

Compassionate Choices
A community-based, statewide organization that provides information and referrals connecting the seriously ill, their loved ones and caregivers with life-affirming resources in their communities. Produces a statewide resource guide which lists resources by county. Western Washington: 300 Elliott Avenue West, Suite 300, Seattle, WA 98119. 888-753-7312

Disabled Person Parking Privileges
Information and applications for temporary disabled parking permits may be obtained in some treatment facilities. A physician's certification of disability is required, and permanent placards require photo identification at local driver licensing offices. Department of Licensing, Disabled Parking, P.O. Box 9030, Olympia, WA 98507. (360) 902-3770; Fax: 360-664-0339

Encore Program (YWCA)
Aquatics exercise for breast cancer survivors. Tacoma: (253) 272-4181

Meals on Wheels
Program of Senior Services of Seattle/King County, 1601 2nd Avenue, Suite 800. Seattle, WA 98101-1579. Fax: 206-448-5756. Delivers 7 to 28 frozen meals weekly to homebound elderly and disabled. Donation requested. Seattle area (206) 448-5767, Shoreline (206) 365-1536, Auburn (253) 931-3016

Lawyer Referral Service
King County Bar Association-sponsored service providing information and referral to local attorneys. Some low-cost or pro bono services may be available. (206) 623-2551

METRO Regional Reduced Fare Permit
A $3.00 permit for discount fares on eight transportation systems throughout the Puget Sound region for people 65 or older or those disabled by cancer or cancer treatment. Requires physician verification. (206) 553-3060

METRO Special Transportation Services Program
If you cannot ride the bus because of financial need or disability, you may qualify for van or taxi service at a 50% reduction. (206) 553-3060

METRO Carpool and VanPool Service
For persons unable to use regular bus transportation in King County. (206) 625-4500. Applications must be signed by a medical social worker or other professional.

Senior Information and Assistance
Advocates put seniors in touch with community resources. Seattle: (206) 448-3110; other locations: (800) 972-9990. www.seniorservices.org

Social Security Disability or Social Security Income
Provides information concerning federal financial assistance. 720 Olive Way, 2nd Floor, Seattle, WA. (800) 772-1213 (7 a.m. to 7 p.m.)

Metro King County ADA Paratransit Program
Provides low-cost, wheelchair-accessible transportation on a pre-scheduled basis, door-to-door. (206) 689-3113

Washington State Assistance
Department of Social and Health Services. Local offices are listed in the blue pages of the Seattle phone book under Washington State Community Service Offices. Provides public assistance and Medicaid coupons to cover the costs of medical treatment, medications, etc., to eligible applicants.

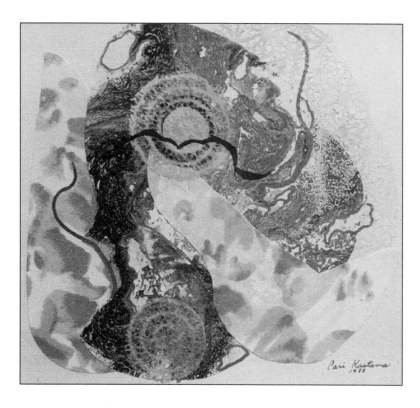

Cari Kastama ❧ *Soft Moon Shadows* ❧ Mixed Media & Collage

20

Resources for Specific Populations

African American Community Services
Center for Multicultural Health
105 14th Avenue, Suite 2C
Seattle, WA 98122
KimTaylor, (206) 461-6900, ext. 231

> *Educational and outreach services:* Covered by the Breast and Cervical Health Program: uninsured or under-insured women, 40 years of age and older, are eligible for screening services and health examinations.

> *Circle of Friends:* support groups that meet at three locations: the Central area, South Seattle and Bellevue.

> *Tele-friend Program:* Adapted from the American Cancer Society Tele-friend program. African American women offer information on cancer issues via telephone and encourage one another to get mammograms and pap tests.

National Black Leadership Initiatives on Cancer
105 14th Avenue, Suite 2C
Seattle, WA 98122
KimTaylor, (206) 461-6900, ext. 231
Shelley Cooper-Ashford, (206) 461-6910
Works in conjunction with the Breast and Cervical Health Program. Outreach services and informational materials on breast cancer prevention and diagnosis.

Sisters Network
8787 Woodway Dr., Suite 4207
Houston, TX 77073
(713) 781-0255
Fax: (713) 780-8998
An African American breast cancer survivors' support group.

Asian American Community Services
International District Community Health Center
416 Maynard Avenue South
Seattle, WA 98104
(206) 461-3235
Covered by the Breast and Cervical Health Program. Uninsured or underinsured women, 40 years of age and older, are eligible for screening services and health examinations.

Hispanic Community Services
Sea Mar Community Health Center
8720 14th Avenue South
Seattle, WA 98108
(206) 762-3730
A breast health outreach program offering educational services and family support groups to Hispanic women with breast cancer in Seattle/King County. Also covered by the Breast and Cervical Health Program: uninsured or under-insured women, 40 years of age and older, are eligible for screening services and health examinations.

American Cancer Society (ACS) Reach to Recovery Program
Spanish language translation and visitation services.
Trinidad Jimenez, (206) 789-7045

Lesbian Community Services
Mary-Helen Mautner Project for Lesbians with Cancer
1707 L St. NW, Suite 500
Washington, DC 20036
(202) 332-5536
Fax: (202) 265-6854

Seattle Lesbian Cancer Project
1122 E. Pike Street, PMB 1333
Seattle, WA 98122
(206) 323-6540
E-mail: slcp@drizzle.com.
A grassroots lesbian organization dedicated to providing education, support services, and accessible lesbian-sensitive health services to all lesbians and their families living with cancer, especially those who are medically underserved. Services include:

- Lesbian Breast and Cervical Health Program: Uninsured or underinsured women, 40 years of age and older, are eligible for free screening services and health examinations.

- Weekly cancer support groups at two locations: Capitol Hill (206) 286-0166, and the North End (206) 363-7608.

- Free massages for lesbian women with cancer.

- Links with other cancer patients for one-on-one support.

- A monthly newsletter.

Seattle Lesbian Resource Center
2214 S. Jackson Street
Seattle, WA 98144
(206) 322-3953
Internet: www.lrc.net
Educational resources for breast cancer patients.

Low-Income Women — Community Services
Breast and Cervical Health Program
(206) 286-0166 or (800) 756-5437 (Community Health Access Program)
Low-income women 40 years of age and older who are uninsured or under-insured are eligible for screening services and health examinations for up to three years at participating clinics. Call the Community Health Access Program for eligibility information and referral to participating clinics.

Chicken Soup Brigade
Delivers meals to the homes of low-income, chronicly or terminally ill women.
To apply, (206) 440-8854

National Cancer Institute's Cancer Information Service
(800) 422-6237
Provides information on local facilities offering low-cost or free mammography services.

Medicare
Consumer Services & Information
(206) 615-2354 or (800) 638-6833
Offers informational brochures on mammograms. Also provides literature on Medicare.

Encore Plus Program
YWCA Health Promotion
1118 5th Avenue
Seattle, WA 98101
(206) 461-4454
Offers mammograms and examination services to women who are low-income and under-insured. Provides educational services to women with breast cancer, as well as access to free exercise classes.

Native American Community Services
Seattle Indian Health Board
611 Avenue South
Seattle, WA 98114
(206) 324-9360/324-8484
Offers primary care on a sliding scale fee basis, and referral services. Also covered by the Breast and Cervical Health Program: uninsured or underinsured women, 40 years of age and older, are eligible for screening services and health examinations.

Women Eligible for Military Services
Madigan Army Medical Center
Ft. Lewis, WA 98433
(253) 968-0975
Offers multidisciplinary services including screening, diagnostic testing and treatment services. Served by the Reach to Recovery program. Also offers education and support services to Bremerton and Whidbey Island Naval Hospitals and McChord and Fairchild Air Force Bases. On-line access to the NCI Cancer Information Service.

GANTS
(360) 491-4590
Ongoing breast cancer support group attended by women of all ages and backgrounds. Welcomes non-military as well as military-eligible breast cancer patients. The group meets at the Family Resource Center at Ft. Lewis, near Tacoma, WA.

Foreign Language Translation Services
American Cancer Society Reach to Recovery Program
800-ACS-2345
Brochures available in various languages on early breast cancer detection, breast self-examination and diagnosis.

Chocolate on my Head

by Kai Leamer

Good news they say,
let's have a look
come down and do a mammogram.
What's that you say?
You've lost my film?
You don't know where,
I've lost my hair, but you don't care.
You shove my breast in anyway,
I'll try not to squeeze too hard.
Hey, wish I could shove yours in there,
let's see how you like it dear!
What? The left one too?
Is it my fault you've lost them whoo!
And so I'm mad as you can see,
I even tell you what I see on those
new mammograms.
Now dear, you know I can't tell you
what I see so let me show you to the door.
I cry, then get mad, I slam the door.
Across the street I go,
Hot chocolate sounds great.
So what if I've given up things that are bad-—
I'm mad!
With no time to spare, I cross the street.
The wind comes up, I fumble with
my chocolate cup, my hat flies
through the air.
I turn to grab my hat, the light turns green
the cars screech to a halt as if in some
Dali scene.
How bizarre, this bald woman dressed in green
chasing a hat with traffic stopped,
should somehow appear more serene.
Chocolate here, chocolate there,
chocolate everywhere.
Amidst the crowd, the hollow stares I dread
a silent tear trickles down.
As I reach up to wipe my tears,
there's chocolate on my head.

21

Western Washington Breast Cancer Treatment Centers

ABERDEEN
Multi Specialty Clinic
East Campus: 915 Anderson Drive
Aberdeen, WA 98520
(360) 537-6391
Inpatient Facility: Grays Harbor
Community Hospital

ANACORTES
Island Hospital
Chemotheraphy/Oncology Dept.
1211 24th
Anacortes, WA 98221-2590
(360) 299-1300, ext.2422

ARLINGTON
North Snohomish County Health
System
330 S. Stillaguamish Ave.
Arlington, WA 98223-1642
(360) 435-2133
Inpatient Facility: Cascade Valley
Hospital

AUBURN
Auburn Regional Center for
Cancer Care
222 2nd St. NE
Auburn, WA 98002
(253) 735-7575
Inpatient Facility: Auburn Regional
Medical Center

BELLEVUE
Overlake Hospital Medical Center
Associates
1035 116th Ave. NE
Bellevue, WA 98004
(425) 688-5220

BELLINGHAM
St. Joseph Hospital Community
Cancer Program
Radiation Oncology Dept.
3217 Squalicum Parkway
Bellingham, WA 98225
(360) 738-6740

BREMERTON
Cancer Services
2520 Cherry Ave.
Bremerton, WA 98310
(360) 792-6885
Inpatient Facility: Harrison Memorial
Hospital

BURIEN
Highline Hospital Cancer Care
Program
16251 Sylvester Rd SW
Seattle, WA 98166
(206) 439-5577

COUPEVILLE
Whidbey General Hospital
Community Cancer Center
101 N Main
Coupeville, WA 98239
(360) 678-5151, ext. 2650

ENUMCLAW
Enumclaw Community Hospital/
Chemotherapy/Oncology Dept.
1450 Battersby Avenue, Box 218
Enumclaw, WA 98022-0218
(360) 825-2505

EVERETT
Providence Medical Center-Everett
Pacific Campus (Radiation Only)
916 Pacific
Everett, WA 98201
(425) 258-7255

FEDERAL WAY
St. Francis Hospital Cancer Care
Center
3409 9th Ave S., Suite 205
Federal Way, WA 98003
(253) 952-7997

OCEAN PARK
North Beach Clinic
21610 Pacific Hwy
Ocean Park, WA 98640
(360) 665-3000

KIRKLAND
Cascade Cancer Center
12303 NE 130th Lane, Suite 120
Kirkland, WA 98034
(425) 899-3181
Inpatient Facility: Evergreen Hospital

LONGVIEW
Peace Health Cancer Center
1614 E. Kessler Blvd./P.O Box 3002
Longview, WA 98632-0302
(360) 414-7572
Inpatient Facility: St. John Medical
Center

MOUNT VERNON
North Puget Sound Oncology
1415 E. Kincaid Street, P.O. Box 1376
Mount Vernon, WA 98273-1376
(360) 428-2146
Inpatient Facility: Skagit Valley
Hospital (Oncology only)
United General Hospital (Radiation
and Medical oncology)

OLYMPIA

Western Washington Cancer
Treatment Center
3920 Capital Mall Dr. SW, Suite 100
Olympia, WA 98502
(360) 754-3934
Inpatient Facility: Columbia Capital
Medical Center

Memorial Clinic
Dept. of Oncology
500 Lilly Rd. NE
Olympia, WA 98506
(360) 456-1122 ext. 8513

PORT TOWNSEND

Jefferson General Hospital
Radiology Oncology Dept.
834 Sheridan
Port Townsend, WA 98368-2443
(360) 385-2200, ext. 3500

PUYALLUP

Good Samaritan Hospital
Chemotherapy/Oncology Dept.
407 14ᵗʰ Avenue SE
Puyallup, WA 98372-0118
(253) 848-6661
Radiology: ext. 1840
Oncology: ext. 2400

RENTON

Valley Medical Center
Oncology Dept.
400 S 43ʳᵈ St.
Renton, WA 98055
(425) 656-4002

SEATTLE

Group Health Cooperative Central
Specialty Center
125 16ᵗʰ Avenue E
Seattle, WA 98112
(206) 326-3111
Inpatient Facility: Virginia Mason
Hospital

Harborview Medical Center
325 Ninth Ave.
Seattle, WA 98104
(206) 731-3913

Fred Hutchinson Cancer Research
Center
1124 Columbia St.
Seattle, WA 98104
(206) 667-5000
Limited experimental treatment
(stem cell transplants). Must be
referred by a physician.

Northwest Cancer Center
1560 N 115ᵗʰ G-16
Seattle, WA 98133
(206) 365-8252
Inpatient Facility: Northwest Hospital

Pacific Medical Center
1101 Madison St.
Seattle, WA 98104
(206) 505-1440
Radiation and Chemotherapy
Oncology
Inpatient Facilities: Providence
Medical Center and Swedish Medical
Center

The Polyclinic
1145 Broadway
Seattle, WA 98104
(206) 329-1760
Inpatient Facility: Swedish Medical
Center

Providence Comprehensive Breast
Center
550 16ᵗʰ Ave, #400-401
Seattle, WA 98122
(206) 320-4800 or 320-4880
Inpatient Facility: Providence Medical
Center

Southwest Tumor Institute
16251 Sylvester Rd SW
Seattle, WA 98166
(206) 386-2626
Inpatient Facility: Highline
Community Hospital

Swedish Tumor Institute – Breast
Care Center
1101 Madison St., Ste. 310
Seattle, WA 98104
(206) 386-3776
Inpatient Facility: Swedish Medical
Center – First Hill

Swedish Tumor Institute – Ballard
1801 NW Market, #207
Seattle, WA 98107
(206) 386-6707
Radiation therapy only

University of Washington Breast
Cancer Specialty Center
1959 NE Pacific Ave
Seattle, WA 98195
(206) 598-4104

Virginia Mason Cancer Center
1100 Ninth Ave
Seattle, WA 98111
(206) 223-6881

SEDRO WOOLLEY
North Puget Oncology
1971 Highway 20
Sedro Woolley, WA 95284
(360) 856-7581
Inpatient facility: United General
Hospital

SEQUIM
Sequim Radiation /Oncology Dept.
615 N 5th
Sequim, WA 98382
(360) 683-9895; fax: (360) 683-0135
Inpatient facility: Olympic Memorial
Hospital

SHELTON
Mason General Hospital Oncology/
Medical Care Facility
901 Mt. View Dr., Building #2
Shelton, WA 98584
(360) 427-7333

TACOMA
MultiCare Hematology/Oncology
Clinic
1003 S 5ᵗʰ St
Tacoma, WA 98405
(253)552-1677
Inpatient Facility: Tacoma General
Hospital

Madigan Army Medical Center
Department of Army
Oncology Services
Tacoma, WA 98431
(253) 968-1055

St. Joseph's Medical Center
Radiation Oncology Dept.
1717 South J Street
Tacoma, WA 98401-2197
(253) 591-6810

VANCOUVER
Southwest Washington Medical
Center
Medical/Oncology Dept.
505 N.E. 87th Ave.
Vancouver, WA 98668
(360) 604-2550
Radiation/Oncology Dept.
400 N.E. Mother Joseph Place
Vancouver, WA 98668
(360) 604-2169

	DIAGNOSTIC				TREATMENT						SERVICES						INFO.	
	Diagnostic Biopsy	Mammography	Ultrasound	Other Breast Imaging	Breast Surgery	Medical Oncology	Inpatient Chemotherapy	Outpatient Chemotherapy	Radiation Therapy	Reconstruction	Financial Counseling	Lymphedema Treatment	Physical Therapy	Nutrition Counseling	Social Services	Support Group	Cancer Education	Genetics Counseling
Aberdeen Multi-Specialty Clinic	✓	✓	✓	✓	✓	✓	✓	✓		✓	✓	✓	✓	✓	✓	✓	✓	✓
Auburn Regional Ctr. for Cancer Care	✓	✓	✓	✓	✓	✓	✓	✓	✓	✓		✓	✓	✓	✓	✓	✓	
Enumclaw Community Hospital	✓	✓	✓		✓	✓		✓		✓	✓		✓	✓	✓	✓	✓	
Everett Clinic	✓	✓	✓	✓	✓	✓	✓	✓	✓	✓	✓	✓	✓	✓	✓	✓	✓	
Evergreen Cancer Center	✓	✓	✓	✓	✓	✓	✓	✓	✓	✓	✓	✓	✓	✓	✓	✓	✓	✓
Group Health Cooperative Central Specialty Center	✓	✓	✓	✓	✓	✓	✓	✓	✓	✓	✓			✓	✓	✓	✓	
Harborview Medical Center	✓	✓	✓		✓	✓	✓	✓	✓	✓	✓	✓	✓	✓	✓			
Harrison Memorial Hospital	✓	✓	✓	✓	✓	✓	✓	✓	✓	✓	✓	✓	✓	✓	✓	✓	✓	
Highline Hospital Cancer Care Program	✓	✓	✓	✓	✓	✓	✓	✓	✓	✓	✓	✓	✓	✓	✓	✓	✓	
Island Hospital		✓		✓	✓		✓	✓		✓	✓		✓	✓	✓	✓	✓	
Jefferson General Hospital	✓	✓	✓		✓		✓	✓				✓	✓	✓	✓	✓	✓	✓
Madigan Army Medical Center	✓	✓	✓	✓	✓	✓	✓	✓	✓	✓		✓	✓	✓	✓	✓	✓	
Mason General Hospital	✓	✓	✓		✓	✓	✓	✓		✓	✓	✓	✓	✓	✓	✓	✓	
North Puget Oncology	✓	✓	✓	✓	✓	✓	✓	✓	✓	✓	✓	✓	✓	✓	✓	✓	✓	
North Snohomish County Health System		✓	✓		✓	✓		✓		✓	✓				✓	✓	✓	
Northwest Cancer Center	✓	✓	✓		✓	✓	✓	✓	✓	✓						✓	✓	
Ocean Beach Hospital	✓	✓	✓		✓	✓		✓	✓	✓	✓	✓	✓	✓	✓	✓	✓	✓
Overlake Hospital Medical Center Associates	✓	✓	✓		✓	✓	✓	✓	✓	✓		✓	✓	✓	✓	✓		
Pacific Medical Center	✓	✓	✓		✓	✓	✓		✓	✓	✓	✓	✓	✓	✓	✓	✓	✓

	DIAGNOSTIC				TREATMENT						SERVICES						INFO.	
	Diagnostic Biopsy	Mammography	Ultrasound	Other Breast Imaging	Breast Surgery	Medical Oncology	Inpatient Chemotherapy	Outpatient Chemotherapy	Radiation Therapy	Reconstruction	Financial Counseling	Lymphedema Treatment	Physical Therapy	Nutrition Counseling	Social Services	Support Group	Cancer Education	Genetics Counseling
Peace Health Cancer Center	✓	✓	✓		✓	✓	✓	✓	✓	✓	✓	✓	✓	✓	✓	✓	✓	
The Polyclinic	✓	✓	✓	✓	✓	✓	✓	✓		✓								
Providence Comprehensive Breast Center	✓	✓	✓	✓	✓	✓	✓	✓	✓			✓	✓	✓	✓	✓	✓	✓
Providence-Everett Medical Center	✓	✓	✓	✓	✓	✓	✓	✓	✓	✓	✓	✓	✓	✓	✓	✓	✓	
Providence/St. Peter's Hosp. Memorial Clinic/Oncology	✓	✓	✓	✓	✓	✓	✓	✓	✓	✓	✓	✓	✓	✓	✓	✓	✓	✓
Puget Sound Cancer Center	✓	✓	✓		✓	✓	✓	✓		✓						✓	✓	
St. Francis Hospital Cancer Care Center	✓	✓	✓		✓	✓	✓	✓		✓	✓	✓	✓	✓	✓	✓	✓	✓
St. Joseph Hospital Community Cancer Prog.	✓	✓	✓		✓	✓	✓	✓	✓	✓	✓	✓	✓	✓	✓	✓	✓	
Southwest Tumor Institute							✓	✓			✓							
Southwest Washington Medical	✓	✓	✓		✓	✓	✓	✓	✓	✓	✓		✓	✓	✓	✓	✓	
Sequim Radiation and Oncology	✓	✓	✓		✓	✓	✓	✓	✓			✓	✓	✓	✓	✓	✓	
Swedish Tumor Institute — Ballard	✓	✓	✓	✓	✓	✓	✓	✓	✓	✓	✓	✓	✓	✓	✓	✓	✓	✓
Swedish Tumor Institute Breast Care Center	✓	✓	✓	✓	✓	✓	✓	✓	✓	✓	✓	✓	✓	✓	✓	✓	✓	✓
Tacoma Multicare Regional Cancer Center	✓	✓	✓		✓	✓	✓	✓	✓						✓	✓	✓	✓
UWMC Breast Care and Cancer Research Center	✓	✓	✓	✓	✓	✓	✓	✓	✓	✓	✓	✓	✓	✓	✓	✓	✓	✓
Valley Medical Center	✓	✓	✓	✓	✓	✓	✓	✓	✓	✓	✓	✓	✓	✓	✓	✓	✓	
Western Washington Cancer Treatment Center	✓	✓	✓		✓			✓	✓	✓			✓	✓		✓		✓
Whidbey General Hospital Community Cancer Center	✓	✓	✓	✓	✓	✓	✓	✓			✓	✓	✓	✓	✓	✓	✓	

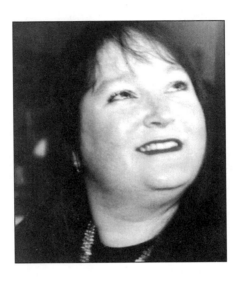

Rebecca Maryatt
Diagnosed: Age 36, 1992

I noticed an enlarged axillary lymph node under my arm in the shower. My internist sent me for a mammogram. It was reviewed, and I was sent to a surgeon. I credit my monthly breast self-exam, a mammogram, and clinical exam along with a wonderful team of doctors and their staffs for saving my life. While it scared me, breast cancer also made me angry. As a result, I have become a breast cancer activist. I tell women to be pro-active. Educate yourself and become involved in the fight. Know your own body. If you can, help someone else. Pass the word along about the importance of early detection. You can survive!

22

Breast Cancer Information: Books, Videos, the Internet, and Beyond

ᏇᎧ

There is nothing quite like having breast cancer to spark one's interest in the subject. Fortunately, the Puget Sound area has some of the best resources for obtaining medical information anywhere in the U.S. These range from bookstores to regional patients' and medical research libraries.

When gathering information on medical topics, books written for laypeople are often a good start. These are available at bookstores and local libraries. The Seattle Public Library has a bibliography on breast cancer available at most branches and at the Downtown Library at 4th and Madison, (206) 386-4636.

The King County Library system, (800) 462-9600, has a medical librarian and a user-friendly computerized bibliography of medical information on Infotrac. You can request information on medical topics and make your own list of recent articles published in popular magazines and some medical journals. Often, you can read the full text of the article right on the screen. The quality of this information varies, but is often excellent.

Several local hospitals have collections of reading materials and tapes for patients. Our region also has a Planetree Library, the ultimate in patient libraries. Planetree is a national organization dedicated to improving the quality of health and hospital care and providing the public with medical information. There are about eight Planetree libraries in the U.S. In a very comfortable setting it has books, audio and video tapes, a computer database, magazines, medical journals, clippings on medical and health topics, and a friendly librarian. Use of materials in the library is free, a copy machine is available, and checkout privileges are obtained by joining

Planetree for a nominal fee. The library is located in Burien just south of Highline Hospital at 16251 Sylvester Rd. SW (206-244-4052). Hours are Tuesday, Thursday, and Saturday 11 am to 5 pm, Wednesday 2-8 pm, and other times by appointment.

For those who wish to obtain the same medical information professionals use, the Pacific Northwest Regional Health Sciences Libraries and Information Center at the University of Washington is also available. Located in the second floor T-wing of the Health Sciences Building on NE Pacific Avenue, it is open to the public. Materials can be used in the library and copied for 10 cents a page. It has most current medical journals, shelved alphabetically by title (free library maps show where). User-friendly databases, including Medline, can be searched by subject, title, author, etc. Medline is a computer searchable database of medical journals and books, which is also available to the public through PubMed on the Internet, www.ncbi.nlm.nih.gov/PubMed/.

An evening class in use of medical libraries and medical databases called "Patient Power" is held at the UW Health Sciences Library every quarter through the Seattle Central Community College Continuing Education Program, call (206) 587-5473, for registration assistance. The Health Sciences Library hours are 7 am to 10 pm most days during the school year, (206) 543-5530.

⑩RESOURCES

This Resource List is made available by the Komen Foundation for your personal benefit. It is not a complete listing of materials available on breast health and breast cancer. Further, the Komen Foundation does not endorse or recommend these publications or make any warranties or representations regarding the accuracy, quality or appropriateness of any of the information contained therein.

Prevention

Women's Cancers: How to Prevent them, How to Treat them, How to Beat them by Kerry McGinn and Pamela Haylock: 1998.

> A team of nurses, a breast cancer survivor and a cancer-care consultant examine the fears, myths and truths about pelvic, uterine, ovarian and rare gynecologic cancers.

Risk Factors

Breast Cancer: Reducing Your Risk (If it Runs in your Family) by M.D. Eades; Bantam Books: 1991.

A handbook containing necessary information to assess one's personal risk and to make necessary changes to maintain optimum health.

Diagnosis

Be A Survivor: Your Guide to Breast Cancer Treatment by Vladimir Lange, M.D.; Lange Productions: 1998.

The book presents a continuum of information for the newly diagnosed breast cancer patient and her partner from diagnosis through recovery. Quotations from breast cancer survivors, questions to ask your physician and informative illustrations provide a comprehensive overview of breast cancer.

Bosom Buddies by Rosie O'Donnell and Deborah Axelrod, M.D., F.A.C.S.; Warner Books: New York, New York, 1999.

The book covers a variety of topics including breast health, screening, risk factors, diagnosis, treatment, follow-up treatment, research and resources. It is written in a humorous yet informative manner, following a question and answer format. Puzzles, songs, jokes, cartoons and a resource list are provided.

Breast Cancer: The Complete Guide by Yashar Hirshaut, M.D. and Peter Pressman, M.D.; Bantam Books: 1996.

Written by a surgeon and an oncologist, this book provides a comprehensive review of the breast cancer experience from diagnosis to treatment, to life after treatment.

Diagnosis Cancer, Your Guide through the First Few Months by Wendy Schlessel Harpham, M.D.; W.W. Norton & Co: 1997.

Written by a physician and past cancer patient who writes from the perspectives of both doctor and patient, this book provides questions to ask during the first few months following diagnosis.

Dr. Susan Love's Breast Book by Susan Love, M.D. with Karen Lindsey; Addison Wesley: Second edition 1995.

> Written by a breast surgeon, this book contains information about breast diseases and beast health. A good resource for every woman, whether or not she has breast cancer.

In Touch With Your Breasts by James Davidson, M.D. and Jan Winebrenner; WRS Publishing: 1994.

> Written in a question and answer format, this book includes questions for women diagnosed with breast cancer as well as women with questions about general breast health. Features a lifelike mini-breast model with two identifiable lumps.

Straight Talk about Breast Cancer from Diagnosis to Recovery: A Guide for the Entire Family by Suzanne W. Braddock, M.D., Jane M. Kercher, M.D., John J. Edney, M.D., and Melanie Morrissey Clark; Addicus Books: 1996.

> Written by a doctor, the book is a guide for the whole family, answering common questions about breast cancer.

The Breast Cancer Companion by Kathy La Tour; Avon Books: 1994.

> A breast cancer survivor combines personal stories with medical information that provides a comprehensive overview.

The Breast Cancer Handbook by Joan Swirsky and Barbara Balaban; Harper Perennial: 1998.

> Written by a clinical nurse specialist and social worker, this book encompasses a step-by-step guide for the woman facing a breast biopsy and diagnosis.

The Breast Cancer Survival Manual by John Link, M.D.; Henry Holt and Company, Inc.: 1998.

> The book is written as a handbook for the newly diagnosed breast cancer patient so that she can get information and be empowered to participate in the decisions regarding her care and treatment. The resource section includes a list of organizations and a discussion of Internet web sites. The author states that he will update the manual through an Internet web page.

The Race is Run One Step At A Time by Nancy Brinker with Catherine McEvily Harris; Summit Publishing Group: 1995.

A down-to-earth resource book explaining medical information and terminology that includes questions to ask your doctor, photographs and a resource section. The book includes the author's own story and the dramatic story of her sister, Susan G. Komen.

Woman to Woman by Hester Hill Schnipper and Joan Feinberg Berns; New York, NY: Avon Books, Inc., 1996. .

Written by two breast cancer survivors, this book is full of positive thoughts, practical advice and tips on how to get through the time from breast cancer diagnosis to treatment. The book covers issues such as finding support, selecting a medical team, treatment tips, treatment decisions, survivorship issues and a comprehensive list of resources.

Treatment

A Woman's Decision: Breast Care, Treatment and Reconstruction by Karen Berger and John Bostwick III, M.D.; Quality Medical Publishing, Inc.: Third Edition 1998.

The book thoroughly explores cancer treatment techniques and medical information. The book details the medical and emotional issues that a woman faces when confronting breast cancer.

Bone Marrow Transplants: A Book of Basics for Patients by Susan K. Stewart; BMT Newsletter: 1995.

Written by patients for patients, with the help of several nurses and doctors, the book describes the procedures and issues surrounding bone marrow transplants.

Breast Implants: Everything You Need to Know by Nancy Bruning; Hunter House: Second edition 1995.

The book provides a comprehensive overview from the perspectives of consumer health advocates, the Federal Drug Administration and the medical community.

Cancer Clinical Trials: Experimental Treatments and How They Can Help You by Robert Finn; Sepastopoal, CA: O'Reilly & Associates, Inc., 1999.

The book provides a good overview of clinical trials for the breast cancer patient and her family or friends. The book details the different phases, ethics, history, types, insurance issues, inclusion/exclusion criteria, administration and evaluation of clinical trials.

Chemotherapy Gives New Meaning to a Bad Hair Day by Eileen Marin; Meltdown International: 1996.

The book balances the emotional issues of a cancer diagnosis with humor. The author focuses on the importance of expressing emotions and using humor to alleviate difficult times.

Coping with Chemotherapy by Nancy Bruning; Ballatine Books, Inc.,1993.

An excellent reference book, including the author's personal experience and commentary from health professionals.

Everyone's Guide to Cancer Therapy by Malin Dollinger, M.D., Ernest H. Rosenbaum, M.D. and Greg Cable; Andrews: Third Edition, 1998.

Good basic information on cancer and treatment options such as chemotherapy, bone marrow transplants, coping and home-care resources.

Healing, A Woman's Guide to Recovery After Mastectomy by Rosalind Delores Benedet, N.P., M.S.N.: 1993.

Written by a nurse practitioner, this is a short and very practical book about mastectomy and recovery.

Living in the Postmastectomy Body: Learning to Live and Love Your Body Again by Becky Zuchweiler, M.S., R.N.; Hartley and Marks Publishers, Inc.: 1998.

The book provides a comprehensive overview of the author's preventive mastectomy experience and the challenges and decisions associated with a mastectomy.

Nutrition for the Chemotherapy Patient by Janet Ramstack, Ph.D. and Ernest H. Rosenbaum, M.D.; Bull Publishing Company: 1990

An informative handbook on chemotherapy drugs and guidelines to prevent common side effects and tips to maintain weight. Includes easy, useful recipes.

The Activist Cancer Patient by Beverly Zakarian; John Wiley and Sons, Inc.: 1996.

Cancer survivor, Beverly Zakarian provides a comprehensive approach for taking charge of one's health including questions to ask your physician, state-of-the-art treatment, drug trials, experimental treatment, journal and database recommendations and support groups.

Follow-up Care and Issues

After Cancer: A Guide to Your New Life by Wendy Schlessel Harpham, M.D.; Harper Collins Publishers, Inc.: 1995.

Written by a physician who is also a cancer survivor, this book addresses the practical issues and the psychosocial elements of recovery after cancer treatment. It provides concrete examples to help survivors deal with emotions.

Beautiful Again: Restoring Your Image and Enhancing Body Changes by Jan Willis; Health Press: 1994.

A good resource for improving self-esteem through the management of a negative physical appearance associated with disability, illness and medical treatment.

Be Prepared: The Complete Financial, Legal and Practical Guide for Living with a Life-Challenging Condition by David S. Landay; 1998.

A guidebook intended to help persons with a life-challenging condition, as well as their families and friends, cope with the financial, legal and practical issues of illness, disability and death.

Dancing in Limbo: Making Sense of Life After Cancer by Glenna Halvorson-Boyd and Lisa K. Hunter; Jossey-Bass Publishers: 1995.

This book offers inspiration, affirmation and straight from the heart talk about the questions that haunt cancer survivors. It is filled with deeply moving insights into the triumphs of cancer survivors who have transformed the threat of death into a celebration of life.

Intimacy: Living as a Woman After Cancer by Jacquelyn Johnson; 1987.

Frank treatment of sexual issues after all types of cancer. Extensive bibliography and resource list included.

Living Beyond Breast Cancer by Marisa C. Weiss and Ellen Weiss; Times Books: 1998.

Written by a doctor, the book is based on the research and clinical results with patients. The book includes information on lymphedema, nutrition, employment, insurance and wills.

Lymphedema, A Breast Cancer Patient's Guide to Prevention and Healing by Jeannie Burt and Gwen White: Publishers Press, 1999.

Written by a patient and physical therapist, the book provides a comprehensive overview of the lymphatic system and lymphedema. It focuses on prevention strategies, standard and unconventional treatment as well as a resource section. It includes anatomy pictures, massage techniques, bandaging and exercise routines. A reference and note section are also included in the back of the book.

To Be Alive, A Woman's Guide to a Full Life After Cancer by Carolyn D. Runowicz, M.D. and Donna Haupt; Diane Publishing: 1998.

Written by an oncologist and breast cancer survivor, this book embodies a guide full of insightful advice.

Upfront—Sex and the Post-Mastectomy Woman by Linda Dackman; 1990.

Written by a single woman with breast cancer, the book explores the emotional aftermath of her mastectomy.

Support For Breast Cancer Patients

Affirmations, Meditations and Encouragements for Women Living with Breast Cancer by Linda Dackman; RGA Publishing: 1991.

Topics span the emotional spectrum of breast cancer diagnosis, treatment and recovery. Included are topics regarding fear of recurrence, anger and living in the present.

Beauty and Cancer, Looking and Feeling your Best by Diane Doan Noyes and Peggy Mellody, R.N.; Taylor Publishing: 1992.

A handbook designed to help women improve their appearance and levels of comfort both during and after cancer therapies.

Breast Cancer: A Family Survival Guide by Lucille M. Penderson and Janet M. Trigg; Bergin and Garvey: 1995.

This book is a helpful guide to detecting breast cancer, dealing with it physically and emotionally, and surviving it. Issues such as insurance, physical changes, family stress, recovery and death are discussed in language for the general reader.

Breast Cancer? Let Me Check My Schedule! by D. Cederberg, D. Davidson, J. Edwards, D. Hebestreit, B. Lambert, A. Langer, C. Masamitsu, S. Snodgrass, C. Stack and C. Washington; Innovative Medical Education Consortium, Inc: 1997.

A compilation of ten professional women meeting the challenges of fitting breast cancer into their very busy lives.

Breast Cancer Survivor's Club: A Nurse's Experience by Lillie Shockney; Windsor House: 1997.

Shockney describes the emotional experience of waiting for diagnosis and treatment, both for herself and her family. Included is a detailed discussion of prosthesis selection and fitting.

Celebrating Life by Sylvia Dunnavant; USFI, Inc: 1995.

This book captures the personal stories and triumphs of African American women in regards to breast cancer.

Examining Myself: the Woman's Story of Breast Cancer Treatment and Recovery by Musa Mayer; Faber and Faber: 1994.

In addition to a detailed account of her breast cancer treatment and reconstructive surgery, Mayer shares her insightful view of survival.

Fine Black Lines: Reflections on Facing Cancer, Fear and Loneliness by Lois Tschetter Hjelmstad; Mulberry Hill Press: 1993.

Through journal entries, poetry, reflective essays and photographs, this book offers poignant insights, realistic optimism and an intimate portrait of courage.

Hope is Contagious—The Breast Cancer Treatment Survival Handbook by Margit Esser Porter; Simon and Schuster, Inc: 1997.

Written by a breast cancer survivor, this book is intended for women who have had or are facing treatment.

Invisible Scars: A Guide to Coping with the Emotional Impact of Breast Cancer by Mimi Greenberg, Ph.D.; Walter & Co.: 1988.

An uplifting book for the newly diagnosed breast cancer patient as well as the woman who has completed her treatment.

Journey Unknown: Focusing on the Emotional Aspects of Cancer, Mastectomy and Chemotherapy by Margaret Phalor Barnhart; Journey Press: 1994.

A collection of poems, thoughts and pictures which express the author's emotions as she experiences cancer, mastectomy and chemotherapy.

Love, Judy: Letters of Hope and Healing for Women with Breast Cancer by Judy Hart; Conari Press: 1993.

The author's personal story combined with a variety of self-support techniques intended to encourage the healing process.

Relaxation and Stress Reduction Workbook by Martha Davis, Elizabeth Robbins Eshelman and Matthew McKay; Fine Communications: Fourth Edition 1998.

A comprehensive, easy-to-follow workbook that explores several techniques to reduce stress, including time management, meditation, assertiveness training, coping skills training, biofeedback, nutrition and exercise.

Spinning Straw into Gold by Ronnie Kaye; Simon and Schuster Trade: 1991.

A counselor shares her personal breast cancer experience and recurrence with wit and understanding. Also included are suggestions for coping and full emotional recovery from breast cancer. An excellent resource for single women.

Straight from the Heart: Letters of Hope and Inspiration from Survivors of Breast Cancer by Ina Yalof; Kensington: 1997.

A collection of 72 letters from breast cancer survivors that share their personal stories.

The Not-so-Scary Breast Cancer Book by Carolyn Ingram, Ed.D. and Leslie Ingram Gebhart, M.A.

Written by two sisters, each diagnosed with breast cancer, the book provides easy to read advice. The authors describe their needs and pitfalls from breast cancer discovery to recovery. The book does not include medical information instead it focuses on support issues. It is a great resource for patients and families desiring something other than the facts, science and medicine of breast cancer.

The Wellness Community Guide to Fighting for Recovery from Cancer by Harold H. Benjamin, Ph.D.; Putnam Books: 1995.

The founder of the Wellness Community shares dozens of well-tasted strategies in which cancer patients can use to maximize the immune system, including visualization, nutrition, exercise and enhanced personal relationships.

Support for Significant Others

Guide for Cancer Supporters by Annette and Richard Bloch; R.A. Bloch Cancer Foundation, Inc: 1995.

Intended for friends or family members of a cancer survivor, this easy-to-follow book provides information on cancer and its treatments as well as ways to support the patient.

Helping Your Mate Face Breast Cancer: Tips For Becoming An Effective Support Partner by Judy C. Kneece, R.N., OCN; EduCare Publishing: 1999.

The book enables the support partner to understand the emotional response of mates, children and themselves; surgical and treatment options to be considered; how to promote the physical and emotional recovery of a mate and how to best manage the role of support partner during the illness.

Man to Man: When the Woman You Love Has Breast Cancer by Andy Murcia and Bob Stewart; St. Martins Press: 1989.

Written by the husband of movie star Ann Jillian, the book provides a helpful account of the authors' reactions to their wives' breast cancer battles.

My Mother's Breast: Daughters Face Their Mother's Cancer by Laurie Tarkan; Taylor Publishing Company: 1999.

The book compiles 16 personal accounts from daughters of mothers who have had breast cancer. The daughters share their feelings of anxiety, loss, fear, courage, inspiration, compassion and joy.

When the Woman You Love Has Breast Cancer by Larry Eiler; Queen Bee Publishing Co.: 1996.

Written from the male perspective, this book describes the experiences and issues faced during his wife's battle with breast cancer.

When Life Becomes Precious by Elise NeeDell Babcock; Bantam Books: 1997.

A comprehensive, easy-to-use handbook that offers uplifting success stories, a resource section and more than 200 tips for friends and loved ones of cancer patients.

Support for Children

Coping When A Parent Has Cancer by Linda Strauss; 1998.

Designed for adolescents, this book provides a complete and frank help for teens of a seriously ill parent.

Moms Don't Get Sick by Pat Brack; Melius Publishing, Inc.: 1990.

Written by a mother and son, this book describes their experience and feelings while the mother was treated for breast cancer.

Once Upon A Hopeful Night by Risa Yaffe; Oncology Nursing Press: 1998.

This book does a wonderful job of helping a parent with cancer explain what is happening to their child. It provides a guide to open communication with their child about the sensitive subject.

Our Family Has Cancer, Too! by Christine Clifford; Pfeifer-Hamilton: 1997.

Clifford shares her personal childhood experiences about her mother's breast cancer as well as her own experiences as a mother with breast cancer.

Paper Chain by C. Blake, E. Blanchard and K. Parkinson; Health Press: 1998.

The illustrated storybook for children provides a general understanding of breast cancer for younger children. The book uncovers the children's feelings of fear and separation as their mother faces surgery, chemotherapy and radiation.

When Eric's Mom Fought Cancer by Judith Vigna; Albert Whitman & Co.: 1993.

This is a storybook for younger children about a mother who undergoes treatment for breast cancer.

Will I Get Breast Cancer? Questions and Answers for Teenage Girls by Carole Vogel; Silver Burdett Press: 1995.

> Written for adolescent girls, this book answers questions on breast health and breast cancer. It also offers practical guidance and comfort to teenagers whose mothers are undergoing breast cancer treatment.

Audio Cassettes

Cancer Survival Toolbox, Building Skills that Work For You developed by the National Coalition for Cancer Survivorship.

> The audio cassettes, designed for cancer survivors, address how to communicate effectively, find information, solve problems, make decisions, negotiate and stand up for your rights. The audio cassettes are available in English and Spanish. (877) 866-5748

Focus on Healing Through Movement and Dance: The Lebed Method of Dance Movement produced by Enhancement, Inc.

> The audio cassette, developed by a breast cancer survivor and physician, is intended for the breast cancer survivor who desires to partake in the healing process as well as regaining strength and movement to the arm. (800) 584-4633

Into the Heart of Breast Cancer: For Women Who Fear and Women Who Have Breast Cancer by Terry Bienkowshi, C.H.

> A series of tapes intended for women that address the emotional, mental and physical aspects of breast cancer. (616) 844-4416

You're Not Alone: Conversations with Breast Cancer Survivors and Those Who Love Them by Voice Arts Publishing Company.

> More than 20 breast cancer survivors share their experiences, well-earned wisdom, humor and advice. (800) 261-1705

Your Present A Half-Hour of Peace by Susie Mantell.

> A guided imagery audio intended for healing, relaxation and wellness. (914) 769-1177

Voices in the Night: A Cancer Companion

A series of tapes intended for the newly diagnosed cancer patient and their partners. Topics include diagnosis, treatment, sexual intimacy and recovery. (800) 268-0009

Video Cassettes

Better Than Before Fitness, Ltd. has designed a rehabilitative/exercise video for breast cancer survivors. The video helps to stretch and strengthen the shoulder, chest, back and abdominal muscles, allowing women to regain full range of motion to those areas affected by breast cancer surgery. www.breastfit.com, (800) 488-8354

Breast Health for Women Over 60, produced by Aquarius Productions, Inc.

The video provides information about mammograms, clinical breast exams and breast self examinations (BSE). Intended for the women over 60, the video demonstrates BSE adaptations for women with arthritis and vision difficulties. (508) 651-2963

Exposure: Environmental Links to Breast Cancer, produced by Francine Zuckerman and Martha Butterfield.

Explores links between breast cancer and the environment. Available in Seattle from Scarecrow Video, (206) 524-8554.

Focus on Healing Through Movement and Dance: For the Breast Cancer Survivor, produced by Enhancement, Inc.

The video, developed by a breast cancer survivor and physician, is intended for the breast cancer survivor who desires to partake in the healing process as well as regaining strength and movement to the arm. (800) 584-4633

For Women Recovering From Breast Surgery, produced by Vickey Pena-Troutman.

A four-series of video tapes focuses on graduated stretching, toning and fat-burning exercises. (800) 454-9889

Lange Productions produces a range of breast health and breast cancer videos, including topics on BSE, mammography and radiation therapy. Videos are regularly updated to include the latest information. (213) 874-4730

Resources on the Internet

The Internet is an amazing source of information about breast cancer. Many excellent web sites are listed on the following pages. Be aware, however, that the accuracy and quality of Internet-derived information can vary greatly from site to site. We suggest that you review and discuss medical information found on the Internet with your health care provider.

Commercial online services often have bulletin boards where cancer survivors regularly provide support and information to each other. Look for these in the Health, Cancer, or Medical sections. Web sites on breast cancer and related topics include:

2 Chicks 2 Bikes 1 Cause (www.2chicks.org)
Information on a bike tour to raise breast cancer awareness in young women, and links to other sites and information on breast health.

American Cancer Society (www.cancer.org)
Nationwide, community-based, voluntary health organization dedicated to eliminating cancer as a major health problem through research, education, advocacy, and service.

American Medical Association (www.ama-assn.org)
Abstracts from the Journal of the American Medical Association (JAMA), nine specialty journals, and the new Women's Health Journal Club.

Breast Cancer Answers (www.medsch.wisc.edu/bca/bca.html)
Responses to questions about all aspects of Breast Cancer provided by trained Cancer Information Specialists using National Cancer Institute-approved resources.

Wisconsin Clinical Cancer Center,
Breast Cancer Information Clearinghouse (www.acor.org)
Current information about breast cancer, including patient-run websites. After reaching the ACOR webpage, click Online Cancer Information and Support.

Breast Care Online (www.medical.informatics.louisville.edu/breast-care/)
From the University of Louisville Medical Informatics Research, this homepage includes much breast cancer patient information provided by cancer centers, links to existing breast cancer-related sites, and other prevention information.

Breast Doctor.Com (www.breastdoctor.com)
This site is designed as an educational tool for breast cancer patients and their families.

178 ᠙ᠥ *Finding Your Way to Wellness*

Cancer Care, Inc. (www.cancercare.com)
Cancer Care, Inc. is staffed by social work professionals offering support services, education and information, referrals and financial assistance.

Cancer Related Links (www.seidata.com/~marriage/rcancer.html)
Comprehensive list of links to many different sites. These include government servers, educational institution servers, cancer institutes and research centers, dedicated cancer links, medical links, journals and newsletters, bone marrow transplants, disease-specific sites, other cancer servers, and alternative and complementary treatments.

CANSearch: A Guide to Cancer Resources on the Internet
(www.access.digex.net/~mkragen/cansearch.html)
Compiled by the National Coalition for Cancer Survivorship (NCCS). The NCCS provides education and advocacy on issues including insurance, employment, and legal rights for people with cancer.

DOD Breast Cancer Decision Guide (www.bcdg.org)
The Department of Defense Breast Cancer Decision Guide is a website developed by the U.S. Department of Defense Breast Cancer Prevention, Education, and Diagnosis Initiative for individuals diagnosed with breast cancer and their families. It provides general information on a variety of breast-related topics.

Edu Care Inc.'s Breast Health and Breast Cancer Network
(www.cancerhelp.com/ed/)
This network has sections for both patient and clinical resources. Patient resources include a woman's guide to breast health services, a supportive partner's questions, a glossary of breast cancer terms and further resources.

Food and Drug Administration (www.fda.gov)
News from the FDA, including the latest and recently approved drugs for treating breast cancer.

Hyperdoc at the National Library of Medicine (www.nlm.nih.gov)
Learn how to connect to comprehensive databases of medical information such as MEDLARS and MEDLINE.

International Cancer Center of the NCI (www.icic.nci.nih.gov)
News and abstracts from the Journal of the National Cancer Institute (JNCI) and other NCI publications. Connect with CANCERLIT, a comprehensive archival file of more than 1,000,000 bibliographic records describing cancer

results published for the past 30 years in biomedical journals, proceedings of scientific meetings, books, technical reports, and other documents.

National Alliance of Breast Cancer Organizations (NABCO) (www.nabco.org) The leading non-profit central resource for information about breast cancer and a network of more than 370 organizations that provide detection, treatment and care to hundreds of thousands of American women. Contains current information about breast cancer, updates on breast cancer-related events and activities, and links to other Internet sites along with NABCO fact sheets and what's new in breast cancer.

National Breast Cancer Coalition (www.natlbcc.org) The NBCC is a grassroots effort in the fight against breast cancer, formed in 1991 to eradicate breast cancer through action and advocacy.

National Cancer Institute (www.cancernet.nci.nih.gov) Learn about ongoing research at NCI. CancerNet is a quick and easy way to obtain cancer information from the National Cancer Institute (NCI). CancerNet lets you request information from the NCI's PDQ database, NCI fact sheets on various topics, and citations and abstracts on selected cancer topics from the CANCERLIT database.

National Lymphedema Network (www.hooked.net/~lymphnet) Information on the prevention and management of lymphedema. The NLN supports research into causes and possible treatments.

OncoLink (www.cancer.med.upenn.edu) Maintained by the University of Pennsylvania as an up-to-date resource on financial resources for cancer patients.

Susan G. Komen Foundation (www.komen.org) and (www.breastcancerinfo.com) A international organization with a network of volunteers working through local affiliates and Komen Race for the Cure® events to eradicate breast cancer as a life-threatening disease by advancing research, education, screening, and treatment.

Washington State Breast and Cervical Health Program (www.fhcrc.org/cipr/bchp/) A Washington State program which provides screening for breast and cervical cancer.

Women's Environment and Development Organization (www.wedo.org)
Website promoting awareness of environmental and economic issues affecting women.

Y-ME National Breast Cancer Organization (www.y-me.org)
This organization provides support and information to anyone who has been touched by breast cancer.

Additional Online Resources

These sites offer additional information on various aspects of breast cancer. The Susan G. Komen Breast Cancer Foundation has no control over the content of these sites.

Alpha Cancer Information Resource
www.alphacancer.com

AMC Cancer Research Center
www.amc.org

American Academy of Family
Physicians
www.aafp.org

American College of Obstetricians
and Gynecologists
www.acog.org

American College of Radiology
www.acr.org

American Medical Women's
Association
www.amwa-doc.org

American Pain Foundation
www.painfoundation.org

American Self Help Clearinghouse
Mentalhelp.net/self help

American Society of Clinical
Oncology
www.asco.org

American Society of Plastic and
Reconstructive Surgeons
www.plasticsurgery.org

Arkansas Department of Health
www.arbreast.com

Ask NOAH about: Cancer
www.noah.cuny.edu

Association of Cancer Online
Resources
www.acor.org

Blood and Marrow Transplant
Newsletter
www.bmtnews.org

Breast Cancer—A Family's Story
www.breastcanceronline.com

Breast Cancer.Net
www.breastcancer.net

Cancer Care
www.cancercare.org

CancerEducation.com
www.cancereducation.com

Cancer News
www.cancernews.com

Cancer Guide: Steve Dunn's Cancer
Information Page
www.cancerguide.org

Cancer Hope Network
www.cancerhopenetwork.org

CancerNet
Cancernet.nci.nih.gov

Cancer Research Foundation of
America
www.preventcancer.org

Cancer Trials
cancertrials.nci.nih.gov

Centers for Disease Control and
Prevention
www.cdc.gov

Centerwatch Clinical Trials Listing
Service
www.centerwatch.com

Department of Defense Breast Cancer
Decision Guide
www.bcdg.org

Department of Health and Human
Services Breast Cancer Area
www.os.dhhs.gov

EduCare
www.cancerhelp.com

FORCE: Facing Our Risk of Cancer
Empowered
www.facingourrisk.org

Gilda Radner Familial Ovarian
Cancer Registry
www.rpci.med.buffalo.edu/
departments/gynonc/group

Health World Online
www.healthy.net

Imaginis.com Breast Health
Specialists
www.imaginis.com

Intercultural Cancer Council
icc.bcm.tmc.edu/home

Lee National Denim Day
www.denimday.com

Living Beyond Breast Cancer
www.lbbc.org

Mautner Project
www.mautnerproject.org

My Image After Breast Cancer
www.proteus1.com/y-me

National Action Plan on Breast Cancer
www.napbc.org

National Alliance of Breast Cancer
Organizations (NABCO)
www.nabco.org

National Asian Women's Health
Organization
www.nawho.org

National Breast Cancer Awareness
Month
www.nbcam.org

National Breast Cancer Coalition
www.natlbcc.org

National Cancer Institute
www.nci.nih.gov

National Center for Complimentary
and Alternative Medicine
nccam.nih.gov

National Coalition for Cancer
Survivorship
www.cansearch.org

National Comprehensive Cancer
Network
www.nccn.org

National Institutes of Health Breast
Cancer Patient Information
wwwicic.nci.nih.gov/pat_home

National Lymphedema Network
www.lymphnet.org

National Women's Health Information
Center
www.4woman.gov

National Women's Health Resource
Center
www.healthywomen.org

Native American Circle
www.mayo.edu/nativecircle

OBGYN.net Latina
Latina.obgyn.net

OncoLink—University of
Pennsylvania Cancer Center
www.oncolink.upenn.edu

Oncology Nursing Society
www.ons.org

SHARE, Self-Help for Women with
Breast or Ovarian Cancer
www.sharecancersupport.org

Sisters Network
www.sisternetworkinc.org

Susanlovemd.com
www.susanlovemd.com

Texas Department of Health, Breast
and Cervical Cancer Control Program
www.tdh.state.tx.us/bcccp

The Gillette Women's Cancer
Connection
www.gillettecancerconnect.org

The Wellness Community
www.wellnesscolumbus.org

Vital Options
www.vitaloptions.org

Y-ME
www.y-me.org

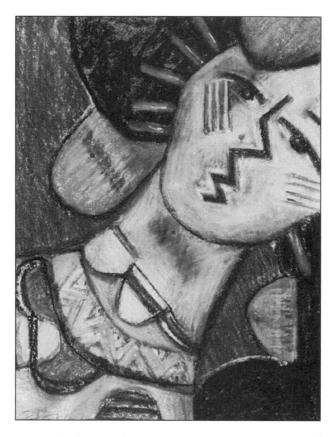

Elizabeth Fischer ❧ *Cancer Warrior* ❧ Pastel

23

Research in Breast Cancer: Hope for the Future

ぞ

Breast Cancer Biology

There is an overriding conviction that success in breast cancer prevention, diagnosis, and treatment lies in a more complete understanding of the cancer cell. Thus, much current research focuses on the biology of normal and malignant breast cells.

Oncogenes are cancer-associated genes which are found in the DNA of all cells and play a role in normal cell growth and differentiation. Oncogenes are usually inactive in normal cells. If they mutate, are amplified, or are "turned on" inappropriately by associated regulatory genes, this can cause the runaway cell growth associated with cancer. An error of DNA replication that results in the activation of an oncogene is like pressing down on the accelerator of a car — it speeds up cell growth and division.

The presence of certain oncogenes is being used to help determine which tumors are likely to recur after surgery, to target treatments, and to predict which treatments are likely to work for a given tumor. HER-2/neu (also called HER-2 or c-erbB-2) is an important oncogene in breast and other cancers. Its presence in a breast cancer is a predictor of tumors that are more aggressive, and less likely to respond to hormone therapy and some forms of chemotherapy. It is also the target of the first FDA-approved biologic therapy used in the treatment of breast cancer, trastuzumab (Herceptin).

Tumor suppressor genes are also cancer-associated genes found in normal DNA. This class of genes acts in the opposite way of oncogenes. These genes are usually turned on in normal cells, suppressing cell growth and division, and aiding in DNA repair. If a mutation or error occurs in a tumor suppressor gene, the affected cell can grow and divide uncontrolled. P53 is one of several tumor suppressor genes associated with breast cancer development.

BRC1 and BRCA2 are two important breast cancer genes associated with a familial tendency to develop breast and ovarian cancer. These genes appear to act as tumor suppressor genes when they are functioning normally, but lose this function when they are mutated in some individuals. An error of DNA replication that results in the deactivation of a tumor suppressor gene is like letting off on the brakes of a car — it speeds up cell growth and division.

Gene Therapy: If we are able to determine the DNA-based changes that have led to the development of a given breast cancer, we have the potential to correct one or more of these DNA mistakes through gene therapy. Early clinical studies are investigating this approach to cancer treatment. One approach is to block inappropriately turned-on oncogenes by "anti-sense" therapy (giving segments of DNA that prevent the gene from functioning). Another approach would include supplying a good copy of a tumor suppressor gene that is not functioning in the tumor cell.

Breast Cancer Genetics

Research into the genetics of cancer is soaring to new heights, and it is now possible to envision the day when the genetic basis of breast cancer will be known, along with mechanisms to correct it. Recent research has targeted two genes responsible for hereditary breast cancer (BRCA1 and BRCA2), which appear to be involved in 5-10 percent of breast cancers. These genes provide tremendous potential for risk assessment and/or early detection of breast cancer. Through genetic engineering, researchers may be able to correct or modify hereditary susceptibility to cancers by transplanting normal copies of genes into cells that have mutated copies of those genes.

Breast Cancer Prevention

In order to make significant strides in breast cancer prevention, the causes of breast cancer need to be better understood. Studies investigating the role of diet, lifestyle factors (stress, exercise), and environmental exposures (radiation, pesticides) will help define the contribution of these factors to breast cancer development. The increased risk (if any) of breast cancer associated with menopausal estrogen replacement therapy will be determined by the large Women's Health Initiative (WHI) study. The anti-estrogens tamoxifen and raloxifene are being studied as breast cancer preventive agents in the National Surgical Breast and Bowel Project's (NSABP) **Study of Tamoxifen and Raloxifene** (STAR) Trial. Researchers are also examining synthetic retinoids (vitamin A-like compounds) like fenretinide, as preventative agents in women at high risk for developing breast cancer.

Breast Cancer Detection and Diagnosis

Until the day that breast cancer can be prevented altogether, early detection of cancer through screening techniques remains our most important tool for maximizing the chance of cure. Mammography is an excellent diagnostic tool in most women, but it lacks sensitivity in the subgroup of patients with dense or irregular breasts. New high-technology diagnostic imaging techniques like Computerized Tomography (CT), Magnetic Resonance Imaging (MRI), and ultrasound are being investigated as possible supplemental tests for imaging "difficult" breasts, to increase the detection of small, hard-to-find tumors at an early stage. Nuclear medicine studies such as MIBI (Miraluma) and PET (Positron Emission Tomography) scans are being studied for a possible role in the diagnosis of breast cancer, as well as in following the response to treatment in patients undergoing chemotherapy.

Many breast imaging centers are now using breast imaging techniques to guide the needle to the tumor. **Stereotactic breast biopsies,** guided by special mammography machines, and ultrasound-guided breast biopsies can direct a biopsy needle to a specific area of abnormality seen on the scan. Guided biopsies can greatly improve the reliability of the tissue sample obtained and result in reduced trauma to the patient.

Breast Cancer Surgery

Breast cancer treatment strategies are constantly evolving, with the goal of achieving maximum benefit for the patient with minimum toxicity and side effects. Breast surgeons have demonstrated through careful clinical trials that reducing the extent of the surgery in appropriately selected breast cancer patients (breast conservation surgery or lumpectomy) can achieve comparable survival results when compared to more extensive surgery (mastectomy).

Reducing the need for axillary lymph node dissection in breast cancer patients is another surgical area of investigation. Although the pathologic lymph node status provides important information that helps in making recommendations about the need for radiation and chemotherapy, the long-term side effects of lymph node removal — lymphedema, nerve injury, and limitations on range-of-motion — can be uncomfortable and occasionally debilitating. Surgeons are currently investigating ways of reducing the number of axillary lymph node dissections performed in breast cancer patients, by using a technique called **sentinel lymph node mapping**. In sentinel lymph node mapping, a small amount of dye and/or radioactivity is injected into the area of the tumor in the breast. The injected substance then travels through the breast lymphatics to the lymph nodes in the armpit (axilla) along the same paths as an errant tumor cell. The surgeon then tracks the path of the dye or radioactivity, and locates the first ("sentinel") lymph node along the pathway.

This lymph node is removed, and the pathologist reviews it for signs of tumor. If this sentinel lymph node is free of tumor, then the chance that nodes farther up the lymph node chain will be involved with tumor is very low. In such a case, the remaining lymph nodes could be left intact, and a full axillary lymph node dissection could be avoided. If the sentinel node contains tumor cells, a full axillary dissection is performed to determine the extent of the spread to the lymph nodes. The success and reliability of sentinel lymph node mapping are presently very dependent on the skill of the surgical team and their ability to correctly identify the sentinel lymph node. Much work remains to be done on perfecting this technique before it can be considered "standard of care."

Systemic Therapy

In the field of medical oncology, many promising new breast cancer chemotherapy treatments are being developed and investigated in clinical trials. Exciting new chemotherapy drugs that have significant activity in breast cancer include paclitaxel (Taxol) and its close relative docetaxel (Taxotere). Vinorelbine (Navelbine), capecitabine (Xeloda), a liposomal form of doxorubicin (Doxil) and gemcitabine (Gemzar) also have demonstrated activity in breast cancer. Many other drugs are in the development phase, or are in early phases of clinical testing.

High-dose chemotherapy treatments are being studied in large clinical trials for patients with aggressive early-stage breast cancer and for advanced disease. Research has shown that tumors may respond better to increased levels of chemotherapy, a so-called "dose-response" level. The dose that can be given to a patient is often limited by the effects of these drugs on the bone marrow. High-dose chemotherapy regimens in breast cancer use chemotherapy doses that are 5-10 times the normal level, in an attempt to eradicate all tumor cells and improve overall survival and cure.

Researchers are testing techniques to stimulate or restore the bone marrow following high doses of chemotherapy, including growth factors (also called cytokines), and bone marrow or peripheral blood stem cell transplantation. These regimens can be toxic and require hospitalization, and the benefits are not yet proven. Early results of recent large, randomized clinical trials have shown mixed results for high-dose chemotherapy/stem cell transplant in both the adjuvant and metastatic cases.

The majority of studies reported to date, most with very early follow-up, have shown no improvement in survival for breast cancer patients who underwent transplantation procedures. A few of these studies do show promise, however, and research continues to try to find the best use of this procedure. Since these studies have not yet proven the benefit of transplantation in breast cancer, it is currently recommended that women considering undergoing high-dose chemotherapy/stem cell transplantation do so in the setting of a clinical trial.

Biotherapy or immunotherapy utilizes components of the immune system, our body's natural defense against infection and cancer, in the treatment program. One problem that has inhibited the development of cancer immunotherapy strategies has been finding "antigens" (targets that stimulate the immune system to respond) that are unique to tumor cells, and that are not found on other normal tissues in the body. Although "tumor-specific" antigens are rare, newly identified "tumor-associated" antigens (proteins that are relatively, but not absolutely, specific to cancer) are being investigated as immunotherapy targets. One of these targets is the oncogenic protein HER-2. Trastuzumab (Herceptin), a monoclonal antibody that targets the HER-2 oncogene, was approved in 1998 for the treatment of metastatic breast cancer.

New techniques have made it possible to produce in the laboratory large quantities of **monoclonal antibodies** directed against certain tumor-associated antigens. These antibodies can be infused into patients, sometimes in combination with drugs or radiation, to target and treat a cancer cell.

Special engineering of monoclonal antibodies has produced **bispecific antibodies** that are directed against both a tumor cell antigen and a protein found on immune system cells. Bispecific antibodies can bring immune system "killer cells" into close contact with the cancer, hopefully resulting in tumor cell death. Researchers are actively investigating **tumor vaccine** techniques, in which patients are injected with combinations of immune-stimulating agents designed to induce a long-lasting immune response against their tumor. Tumor vaccination techniques usually target tumor antigens (like HER-2) found on the cell surface. Tumor vaccines will probably be shown to work best for treating microscopic amounts of breast cancer cells to prevent the disease from recurring.

Bisphosphonates. These drugs prevent the breakdown of bone by osteoclasts — cells whose job it is to regulate normal bone remodeling and growth, but which can also be stimulated by tumor cells to enable cancerous spread within the bone. Alendronate (Fosomax) is an oral drug in this class commonly used to treat osteoporosis in the U.S. Its close relative, pamidronate (Aredia), is a more potent intravenous formulation which has demonstrated efficacy in preventing complications and decreasing pain in women with bone metastases from breast cancer. Clodronate, an oral agent that is less potent than pamidronate, is available in Canada and Europe. Bisphosphonates don't directly target tumor cells but, by inhibiting the osteoclasts, they can delay or potentially prevent spread of tumor in the bones. Large-scale studies are about to begin which will evaluate whether early use of this class of drugs can actually prevent bone metastases from occurring in the first place.

Anti-Angiogenesis Agents. Researchers are trying to understand how cancer cells spread to healthy tissues, a process called metastasis. A cancer cell must recruit new blood vessels into the area of metastasis in order to continue to receive enough nutrients as the tumor enlarges. Cancer cells secrete substances that stimulate the development of new blood vessels, a process called **angiogenesis.** Scientists are studying ways of halting this blood vessel development with drugs called angiogenesis inhibitors in the hope that it will prevent cancers from growing and spreading.

Selective Apoptosis Anti-Neoplastic Drugs (SAANDS). Apoptosis, or "programmed cell death," is a process by which tumor cells die following exposure to chemotherapy and radiation therapy. All cells in our body are capable of undergoing apoptosis when sent appropriate signals, and our body uses this process in the everyday upkeep and turnover of normal tissues. Scientists are working to understand the substances that can stimulate and inhibit this complicated process of cell death. With a better understanding of apoptosis, it may some day be possible to turn on cell death signals specifically in tumor cells.

Drug-Resistance Genes. Breast cancer is often very treatable, but once it has begun to spread, it frequently becomes resistant to chemotherapy drugs. A previously effective treatment can become ineffective as some of the tumor cells survive by finding a way to overcome the toxicity of the drug. Scientists are just beginning to understand how cancer cells manage to survive chemotherapy exposure and develop resistance to chemotherapy. One type of drug resistance is called **multi-drug resistance** (MDR), in which cancer cells become unresponsive to a variety of chemotherapy drugs. The MDR gene produces a protein pump that, when activated, pumps chemotherapy back out of the cancer cell into the surrounding tissue. A number of drugs that inhibit this pump ("MDR inhibitors") are being used in clinical trials to fight this resistance.

Summary

Breast cancer, the most frequently diagnosed cancer in American women, is a complex and devastating disease. Thanks to exciting research advancements in the past decade, we have achieved a better understanding of breast cancer. As a result, we have made strides toward improving breast cancer prevention, diagnosis and treatment strategies. Although the future is promising, we have a long way to go before we are able to eradicate breast cancer in this country. The surest way to achieve success in our quest for a cure for the disease is to foster and ensure funding for broad-ranging research, from basic laboratory work at the cellular level to clinical trials in breast cancer patients.

⊚RESOURCES

National Cancer Institute/Cancer Information Service
1-800-4-CANCER

National Cancer Institute Clinical Trials Website
www:cancernet.nci.nih.gov

CenterWatch
Listing of clinical trials
www.CenterWatch.org

National Library of Medicine's Clinical Trials Database
www.clinicaltrials.gov

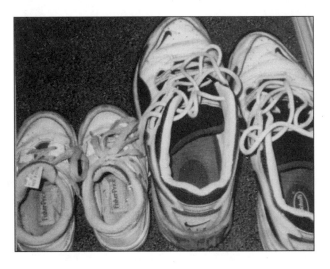

Joan Bowman ❧ *Generations Racing for the Cure* ❧ Photograph

24
Advocacy; Getting Involved

૪ઽ

After a diagnosis of breast cancer, many women have the desire to volunteer or get involved in some type of breast cancer advocacy. Often, families and friends of breast cancer survivors have the same impulse. This can be especially empowering for individuals and help them feel more positive about their own personal experience.

Volunteering

Volunteering at your local hospital or one of the breast cancer organizations in your area is one way to get started. Budgets are often very limited, and there is usually a great need for assistance in clerical work or patient contact. Some organizations require survivors to be out of treatment for at least a year before beginning volunteer work. This helps allow patients plenty of time to regain strength and energy after their treatment and before committing to a new routine or schedule.

A healthy way to get involved is to take part in local "fun" runs/walks and annual events that support breast cancer programs. Being part of a team effort and assisting in a common goal can be very personally satisfying. The Puget Sound Affiliate of the Susan G. Komen Breast Cancer Foundation has an annual Komen Race for the Cure®. You can call the hotline at (206) 667-6700 or contact their website at http://www.seattleraceforthecure.org for more information.

Patient Advocacy

Many organizations, both local and national, help educate women at risk for breast cancer, screen for early detection and/or support breast cancer survivors. As an advocate, your involvement could assist in focusing and assessing concerns within the programs. Specific organizations that are active in representing the breast cancer patient/survivor's viewpoint are NABCO (National Alliance of Breast Cancer Organizations), American Cancer Society, Cancer Care, the Komen Foundation, the National Breast Cancer Coalition and Y-ME. See below for contact information.

Political Advocacy

Contacting your local or state elected officials is the most effective way to take part in a national movement. A national organization that was created to help influence change politically is The National Breast Cancer Coalition. It was developed to encourage women with breast cancer to help improve funding access for better screening, diagnosis and treatment for all women. It has made great strides in creating opportunities for breast cancer survivors to influence and offer input into research, clinical trials, and national policy.

National Organizations

The Susan G. Komen Breast Cancer Foundation and Komen Race for the Cure®
5005 LBJ Freeway, Suite 250
Dallas, TX 75244
(972) 855-1600 or 800-I'M-AWARE

National Alliance of Breast Cancer Organizations
9 East 37th Street, 10th Floor
New York, NY 10016
(888) 806-2226

National Breast Cancer Coalition
1707 L Street NW, Suite 1060
Washington, DC 20036
(202) 296-7477

Y-ME National Breast Cancer Organization
212 W Van Buren St, Fifth Floor
Chicago, IL 60607
(800) 221-2141

Local Organizations

The Susan G. Komen Breast Cancer Foundation
Puget Sound Affiliate
1900 N. Northlake Way, Suite 237
Seattle, WA 98103
(206) 633-0303
sgk@pskomen.org
www.komenseattle.org

American Cancer Society
David Allen, Public Issues Director, Northwest Division
1551 Broadway, Suite 200
Tacoma, WA 98402
(800) 729-3880 or (253) 272-5767

For volunteer opportunities at local hospitals, please see listings in the phonebook and ask to speak to Volunteer Services.

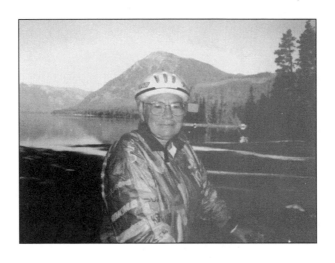

Bonnie Wegner
Diagnosed: 1978

I am now 70 years old. I had a mastectomy 21 years ago. As a long-term survivor, do I ever worry? The answer is yes. I found the lump during a self-exam, and with my head ringing, I raced to the physician's office. The answer at that time was a mastectomy — the sooner, the better. I have always been active: running, cycling and doing triathlons. I wondered what my asymmetric form was going to mean. One of those things meant leaving the prosthesis at home — there are enough things chafing me during a triathlon or running. The surprise is that I've had young men running next to me saying, "Way to go!" My attitude is, "Okay, this has happened, now let's get on with life." It does make you think, and the simple things in life take on a new meaning — running in the rain, biking on a hot day, and the sound of children playing.

"Carpe diem. It's time to enjoy!"

25

Glossary: Important Definitions

This glossary is used with the permission of Clo Wilson-Hashiguchi, author of Stealing the Dragon's Fire.

Adjuvant Treatment: Medical treatment for breast cancer given following surgery or radiation to prevent any further growth of cancer in the body, either at the primary site or elsewhere in the body.

Alopecia: Partial or complete hair loss.

Aneuploid: An abnormal number of chromosomes in cancer cells.

Autologous Bone Marrow Transplant: A procedure in which a patient's own bone marrow is removed (by extracting it with a needle from the hip bone), then stored and later returned to the same person's body after chemotherapy.

Axillary Lymph Nodes: Lymph nodes under the arm.

Benign: Not cancerous.

Biopsy: The surgical removal of a small amount of body tissue so that it can be studied under a microscope.

Biological therapy: The use of biological agents to affect a person's immune system and assist in fighting disease.

Blood Count: The result of an examination of a blood specimen in which the white blood cells, red blood cells, and platelets are counted to determine the balance and number of these elements in the blood.

Bone Marrow: The soft, fatty substance filling the cavities of bones; where blood cells are made.

Breast Reconstruction: Surgery performed to recreate the breast mound, as well as the nipple and areola (dark circle surrounding the nipple), following a mastectomy. A choice is sometimes offered to the patient to have it done at the same time as the mastectomy, or, more frequently, at a later date - often within a year or two. Some reconstruction is performed years after the original surgery.

BSE (Breast Self-Examination): A method used by women to become familiar with the normal appearance and feel of their breast tissue so that if a change occurs it will be detected early. It should be done monthly.

Calcification: *See Microcalcification.*

Cancer: A general term for over 100 diseases in which abnormal cells grow uncontrollably and invade normal cells. They then metastasize, or spread, to other parts of the body.

Carcinogen: Any substance that causes cancer or promotes its growth. For instance, tobacco, asbestos, and some pesticides (such as DDT) are all known carcinogens.

Carcinoma: A cancer that develops in the covering or lining tissues of body organs.

Carcinoma in Situ: The earliest stage of cancer, before the tumor has spread or grown significantly, and is still confined to the local area. Pre-invasive.

Chemotherapy: The treatment of disease by chemical drugs. For breast cancer treatment, some of the more common chemotherapy drugs are cyclosphosphamide (Cytoxan), 5-Fluorouracil (5-FU), doxorubicin (Adriamycin), methotrexate, paclitaxel (Taxol), and docetaxel (Taxotere).

Clinical Trial: A research study that involves people and tries to answer specific questions and find better ways to prevent, diagnose or treat cancer.

Combination Chemotherapy: Treatment with the use of two or more chemicals to achieve the most effective result. Examples of combinations used for breast cancer treatment are: CMF (Cytoxan + Methotrexate + 5-Fluorouracil) and CAF (Cytoxan + Adriamycin + 5-Fluorouracil).

Control Arm: The group of patients in a clinical trial that receives the standard or most commonly accepted treatment.

Cooperative group: An organized group of oncologists from a number of hospitals or clinics who perform clinical studies.

Cyst: An abnormal, sac-like structure that contains liquid or semi-solid material. It may be benign or malignant.

Diagnosis: The process of identifying a disease by its characteristic signs, symptoms, and laboratory findings.

Estrogen: One of the female hormones that maintains the monthly menstrual cycle.

Estrogen Receptor (ER) Assay: A test that determines if the breast cancer in a particular patient is stimulated by estrogen.

Excisional Biopsy: Removal of a suspicious lump in entirety through an incision.

Genes: A hereditary unit. Genes are composed of DNA and found in a specific location on a chromosome.

Grading: A description or classification of a cancerous cell or tumor according to its appearance and growth. Grade I malignancies are more differentiated, which is the most favorable diagnosis; Grade III are the least differentiated, which is the less favorable diagnosis. (See also "Poorly-differentiated cells" and "Well-differentiated cells.")

HER-2 Oncogene: A specific rapid-growth gene found in 30 percent of breast cancers. Also called HER-2/neu and c-erbB-2.

Hickman Catheter: An intravenous tubing which is surgically inserted into a large vein near the heart. The end is tunneled under the skin and pulled out of an opening through the chest, then covered with a removable rubber cap. Medications, fluids, and blood products are inserted through the tubing.

Hormone: A chemical substance produced by glands that affects other tissues in the body.

Hormone Therapy: Treatment of cancer by removing, adding, or blocking hormones that affect the tumor's growth.

Hospice: A program of caring for patients who are dying and the people who support them, with a focus on improving the quality of life.

Hyperplasia, Atypical: Abnormal cell growth.

Imagery: Visualization or use of mental images that come to conscious awareness in a deeply relaxed state to motivate the body's healing.

Immune System: The body's defense system.

Immunotherapy: Therapy that triggers the body's own defense system to control or kill cancer cells.

Incisional Biopsy: Removal of a section of a suspicious lump through an incision. The section is then sent to a laboratory for analysis.

Infiltrating Cancer: *See Invasive Cancer*

Informed Consent: The process by which a person learns about a study treatment, tests, and their possible benefits and risks *before* deciding whether or not to participate.

In Situ: Cancer confined to the local area, pre-invasive. *See Carcinoma in Situ.*

Interferon: A natural chemical made by the body to help fight infections, used in immunotherapy.

Intraductal: Contained within a duct.

Intravenous (IV): The infusion of drugs or fluids through the veins.

Invasive Cancer (Infiltrating Cancer): Cancer cells that have penetrated surrounding normal tissue.

Investigational New Drug (IND): A drug allowed by the FDA to be used in clinical trials but not approved for commercial marketing or general use.

Lats Flap (Latissimus Dorsi Flap): A breast reconstruction procedure in which skin and a piece of muscle from below the shoulder blade area are tunneled under the skin to help form a new breast mound.

Linear Accelerator: An X-ray machine that delivers external radiation therapy, commonly used for radiation treatment of breast cancer.

Lobular: Having to do with the lobules of the breast.

Lobular Carcinoma in Situ: Abnormal cells within the lobule that do not form lumps. Can serve as a marker of future cancer risk.

Lobules: Parts of the breast capable of making milk.

Localized: A cancer confined to the site origin, without evidence of spread.

Lumpectomy: The removal of a cancerous breast lump without the removal of the entire breast. Usually followed by several weeks of radiation treatment.

Lymphatic Vessels: Vessels that carry lymph, a protein-rich fluid that travels between lymph nodes.

Lymphedema: The swelling of an arm or leg caused by an obstructed lymphatic vessel. A possible side effect seen following surgical removal of the lymph nodes.

Lymph Nodes: Glands throughout the body that contain lymphocytes; an important part of the immune system.

Lymphocytes: White blood cells that produce antibodies to kill foreign organisms and cancer cells.

Malignant: Cancerous, as opposed to benign.

Mammogram: Low-dose X-ray used to screen for and diagnose breast cancer.

Margins: The strip of apparently normal surrounding tissue removed with a cancer or biopsy specimen.

Markers (Tumor Markers): Chemicals in the blood that are produced by certain cancers. CA27.29 (CA 15-3) and CEA are common breast cancer markers.

Mastectomy: Surgical removal of the breast as a treatment for breast cancer.

Metastasis: Spread of cancer from one organ to another, usually through the bloodstream or lymphatic system.

Metastasize: To spread to a distant site.

Microcalcification (Calcification): Tiny calcium deposits found in breast tissue, sometimes signaling the presence of breast cancer. Usually detected only by mammogram.

Mitosis: The process of cell reproduction or division.

Modified Radical Mastectomy: The most common type of mastectomy performed today. The breast and some of the underarm lymph nodes are removed, while the chest muscles are left intact.

Mortality Rate: The rate at which people die as a result of a particular cause in a given population.

MRI (Magnetic Resonance Imaging): A machine that creates an image of the body by making a magnetic field and radio waves.

Mutation: The process in which a gene changes.

NCI (National Cancer Institute): A highly regarded federally funded research center in Bethesda, Maryland, that conducts basic and clinical research on new cancer treatments and supervises clinical trials of new treatment throughout the United States.

Needle Biopsy: Removing tissue from a suspicious area by inserting a needle in a tumor and withdrawing cells through it.

Neoplasm: A new abnormal growth, either benign or malignant.

Nuclear Grade: An estimation of the aggressiveness of the cancer by the appearance of the cell's nucleus under the microscope.

NSABP (National Surgical Adjuvant Breast/Bowel Project): A large cooperative group composed of research and clinical physicians who have formed to study new treatments.

Oncogenes: Tumor genes that can transform normal cells into malignant cells.

Oncologist: A physician who specializes in cancer therapy.

Oncology: The study of cancer.

Open Biopsy: A surgery to obtain tissue for examination under the microscope.

Palliative: A treatment to relieve symptoms but not cure the condition.

Palpation: An examination by feeling an area to detect abnormalities.

Pathologist: A physician who specializes in examining tissues under a microscope and diagnosing diseases.

PCA (Patient-Controlled Analgesia): Use of a preprogrammed intravenous pump that delivers a set dose of pain medicine when the patient pushes a button.

PDQ (Physician Data Query): A computer service sponsored by the National Cancer Institute which provides up-to-date medical information on current cancer treatment.

Placebo: A substance with no therapeutic value.

Platelet: A type of cell in the blood that helps it to clot.

Poorly-differentiated (Undifferentiated) Cells: Abnormal cells that lack specialization in function and structure, usually indicating rapidly growing cancer.

Port (Port-A-Cath): A small disc with a soft diaphragm that is surgically placed just below the skin in the chest or abdomen, connecting to tubing which is inserted in a large vein to the heart. Drugs and fluids can be inserted directly into the body via the port without multiple punctures of the veins.

Primary Tumor: The site where a cancer originally began.

Progesterone: One of the female hormones that prepares for conception and performs other functions before and during pregnancy. Certain synthetic forms of the hormone are used in cancer treatment.

Progesterone Receptor (PR) Assay: A test that determines if the breast cancer in a particular patient is stimulated by progesterone.

Prognosis: Expected or probable outcome.

Promoters: Factors that encourage the development of cancer but do not start the process.

Prophylactic Subcutaneous Mastectomy: Removal of all breast tissue beneath the skin and nipple to prevent future breast cancer.

Prosthesis: An artificial replacement for an absent body part.

Protocol: A carefully designed and written cancer treatment plan.

Radiation-Absorbed Dose (RAD): A measure of radiation. One chest X-ray equals one tenth of a RAD.

Radiation Oncologist, Radiotherapist: Two names for a physician who specializes in the use of radiation to treat cancer.

Radiation Therapy: The treatment of cancer using high-energy X-ray.

Radical Mastectomy (Halsted's): The removal of the entire breast along with underlying muscle and the lymph nodes of the armpit. The result is a significant disfigurement of the patient.

Radiologist: A doctor who specializes in imaging studies such as X-rays, CT scans, MRI, and ultrasounds. Radiologists also perform the needle biopsy and wire localization procedure.

Recurrence: A return of cancer in the original site or another location.

Red Blood Cells: Cells in the blood that carry oxygen to the tissues and take away carbon dioxide.

Regression: Cancer that has shrunk due to therapy. In a complete regression, all tumors disappear. In partial regression, some tumor remains.

Remission: Partial or complete disappearance of detectable disease.

Second Opinion: Recommendation from a doctor other than the treating physician.

Side Effect: A secondary effect from the treatment.

Silicone: Synthetic material used in breast implants because of its flexibility and durability.

S-Phase Fraction: The percentage of cancer cells that are in a specific stage (the synthesis phase) of division in the cell cycle. A high SPF number means that the cells are dividing rapidly and the tumor is growing fast.

Staging: The determination of the extent of cancer growth and spread.

Stereotactic Needle Biopsy: A procedure which uses a needle guided into place by computer to obtain a biopsy specimen of a breast change seen on mammography.

Stomatitis: A side effect of chemotherapy that inflames the whole body, usually using drugs.

Tamoxifen: A hormone therapy commonly used to treat both early and advanced stage breast cancer.

T-cell: One of the two major types of lymphocytes that are a part of the body's immune system.

Terminal: Ending in death; fatal.

Tissue Expander: A breast implant that is placed under the chest muscle. The chamber is slowly expanded with weekly injections of salt water through the skin to a port that opens into the chamber. Expanders are used in breast reconstruction, to slowly stretch the chest muscle.

TNM Classification: A system to classify cancers by the size of the tumor (T), lymph node involvement (N), and distant metastasis (M), whether it has spread to other sites in the body.

TRAM Flap (Transverse Rectus Abdominus Myocutaneous Flap): A technique for reconstructing the breast by tunneling abdominal muscle, skin, and fat under the skin to make a new breast mound.

Tumor: A swelling, lump, or mass of tissue which can be either benign or malignant.

Tumor Marker: Chemicals in the blood that are produced by certain cancers.

Undifferentiated Cells: *See Poorly-differentiated cells.*

Well-differentiated Cells: Cancer cells that look similar to normal cells from the same organ; usually a less serious cancer.

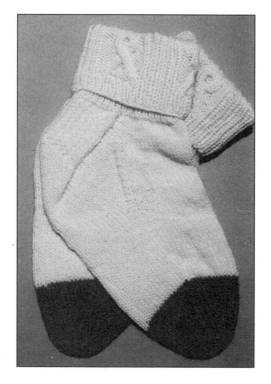

Kendra Elin Aubin
When My Feet Are Warm I Can Face Anything ✌ Hand-Knit Socks

Index

5-fluorouracil (5-FU) 52

Acupuncture 84, 86
Adriamycin (doxorubicin) 52
    side effects 53
Adjuvant therapy 36, 51-58
Advocacy, breast cancer 193-194
African Americans, resources for 149-150
Alendronate (fosamax)
for prevention of osteoporosis 124, 190
Alternative treatments 83-87
Anastrozole (arimidex) 54
Anti-angiogenesis agents 190
Antiestrogens
    see raloxifene
tamoxifen
toremifene
Aredia (pamidronate) 54, 190
Arimidex (anastrozole) 54
Arm swelling (lymphedema) 71-72
Aromatase inhibitors 54
Asian Americans, resources for 150
Audiovisual materials on breast cancer 175-176
Axillary lymph node dissection 40

Basic Health Plan 129
Bellergal for hot flashes 120
Biopsy 18
    sentinel lymph node 40-41

Index of "Wall Of Hope" Survivors

Index of Art And Artists

Notes